Fast Facts: Inflammatory Bowel Disease

Second edition

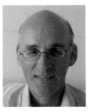

David S Rampton DPhil FRCP
Centre for Adult and Paediatric Gastroenterology
Institute of Cellular and Molecular Science
Barts and The London, Queen Mary School of Medicine
and Dentistry, London, UK

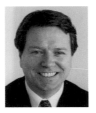

Fergus Shanahan MD
Alimentary Pharmabiotic Centre
Department of Medicine
University College Cork and Cork University Hospital
Cork, Ireland

Declaration of Independence
This book is as balanced and as practical as we can
make it. Ideas for improvement are always welcome:
feedback@fastfacts.com

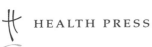

HEALTH PRESS

Fast Facts: Inflammatory Bowel Disease
First published October 2000
Second edition January 2006

Text © 2006 David S Rampton, Fergus Shanahan
© 2006 in this edition Health Press Limited
Health Press Limited, Elizabeth House, Queen Street, Abingdon,
Oxford OX14 3LN, UK
Tel: +44 (0)1235 523233
Fax: +44 (0)1235 523238

Book orders can be placed by telephone or via the website.
For regional distributors or to order via the website, please go to:
www.fastfacts.com
For telephone orders, please call 01752 202301 (UK), +44 1752 202301 (Europe),
1 800 247 6553 (USA, toll free) or +1 419 281 1802 (Americas).

Fast Facts is a trademark of Health Press Limited.

A CIP record for this title is available from the British Library.

ISBN 1-903734-55-X

Rampton DS (David S)
Fast Facts: Inflammatory Bowel Disease/
David S Rampton, Fergus Shanahan

Medical illustrations by Dee McLean, London, UK.
Typesetting and page layout by Zed, Oxford, UK.
Printed by Fine Print (Services) Ltd, Oxford, UK.

Printed with vegetable inks on fully biodegradable and
recyclable paper manufactured from sustainable forests.

Low emissions
during production

Low
chlorine

Sustainable
forests

Glossary of abbreviations

5-ASA: 5-aminosalicylates

ASCA: anti-*Saccharomyces cerevisiae* antibody

ATI: antibodies to infliximab

CARD15: caspase-activating recruitment domain (formerly known as *NOD2*)

CDAI: Crohn's Disease Activity Index

CMV: cytomegalovirus

Cox: cyclo-oxygenase

CT: computed tomography

ERCP: endoscopic retrograde cholangiopancreatography

ESR: erythrocyte sedimentation rate

fMLP: formyl–methionyl–leucyl–phenylalanine

G6PDH: glucose-6 phosphate dehydrogenase

HACA: human antichimeric antibodies, now known as ATI

HLA: human leukocyte antigen

IBD: inflammatory bowel disease

ICAM-1: intercellular adhesion molecule

IFN: interferon

IL: interleukin

MAP: mitogen-activated protein

MHC: major histocompatibility complex

6-MP: 6-mercaptopurine

MRI: magnetic resonance imaging

NF: nuclear transcription factor

NF-κB: nuclear [transcription] factor κB

NOD2: old name for *CARD15*

NOS: nitric oxide synthase

NSAIDs: non-steroidal anti-inflammatory drugs

pANCA: perinuclear antineutrophil cytoplasmic antibody

PPAR: peroxisome-proliferator-activated receptor

PPD: purified protein derivatives (prepared from *Mycobacterium tuberculosis* for the Mantoux test, which indicates past or present exposure to tuberculosis)

SeHCAT: ^{75}selenium-labeled homocholic acid taurine

SLE: systemic lupus erythematosus

^{99}Tc-HMPAO: ^{99}technetium-labeled hexamethyleneamine oxime

TGF: transforming growth factor

Th1: T-helper lymphocyte

TNF: tumor necrosis factor

6-TPMT: 6-thiopurine methyltransferase

VIP: vasoactive intestinal polypeptide

Introduction

Inflammatory bowel disease (IBD) comprises two idiopathic chronic relapsing and remitting inflammatory disorders of the gastrointestinal tract: ulcerative colitis and Crohn's disease. Ulcerative colitis affects only the colon and rectum, while Crohn's disease may involve any part of the digestive tract from mouth to anus.

Over recent decades, the incidence of IBD, particularly Crohn's disease, has been steadily increasing; it now affects more than 2 in every 1000 people in Europe and the USA. Onset is most common in early adulthood, and the chronic waxing and waning nature of ulcerative colitis and Crohn's disease means that together they represent a substantial burden of sickness, not only in hospital clinics and wards, but also in the community. Because of the wide-ranging effects of IBD, multidisciplinary care of affected patients, both within and outside hospital, is essential.

This revised and updated edition of *Fast Facts: Inflammatory Bowel Disease* outlines the etiopathogenesis, presentation, complications, investigation and treatment of ulcerative colitis and Crohn's disease for the non-specialist. We hope that the book will be useful for doctors (particularly primary care physicians and hospital doctors in training), nurses, stoma therapists, dieticians, psychologists, counselors, social workers and other professionals involved in the care of patients with IBD. Medical students should also find it helpful.
Most importantly, perhaps patients with IBD may benefit from reading this overview of their chronic illness.

Although the cause of IBD remains unknown, increasing epidemiological and laboratory data suggest that it results from a genetically determined, inappropriately severe and/or prolonged mucosal inflammatory response to unidentified environmental factor(s), such as dietary or intestinal microbial products (Figure 1.1).

Epidemiology

Incidence and prevalence figures for ulcerative colitis and Crohn's disease are shown in Table 1.1. Both diseases are more common in the Western world than in Africa, Asia or South America. However, the incidence of IBD seems to increase in developing countries as they become more westernized: this phenomenon may be due to enhanced sanitation, vaccination and altered age at exposure to enteric infections.

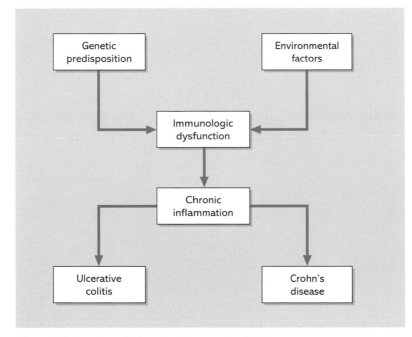

Figure 1.1 Overview of the etiopathogenesis of IBD.

TABLE 1.1

Incidence and prevalence of IBD in the Western world

	Ulcerative colitis	Crohn's disease
Incidence (new cases/100 000 population/year)	10	7
Prevalence (cases/100 000 population)	150	100

In the West, the incidence of Crohn's disease in particular has risen over the last 40 years, though it may now have leveled off.

Both diseases are slightly more common in women and show a bimodal age distribution, with a major peak at 20–40 years of age and a lesser one at 60–80 years. Jewish and Asian people resident in the USA and UK are more likely to be affected by IBD than those living in Israel and Asia, respectively, suggesting that environmental factors are a likely cause. There is no association with social class, but smoking is much more common in patients with Crohn's disease than in those with ulcerative colitis.

Cause

Genetic and other predisposing factors may differ between ulcerative colitis and Crohn's disease.

Genetic factors. Crohn's disease and ulcerative colitis are likely to be related, heterogeneous, polygenic disorders; there is no single Mendelian pattern of inheritance. The genetics of IBD are currently under intense investigation: the findings will have major implications for our understanding of the etiopathogenesis of the disease and for improving its treatment. Genetic factors appear to be more important in Crohn's disease than in ulcerative colitis (Table 1.2).

Ethnic and familial factors. IBD is more common in Ashkenazi than Sephardic Jews, and in North American whites than blacks. The risk of

TABLE 1.2

Genetic factors in the etiology of inflammatory bowel disease

Factor	Ulcerative colitis	Crohn's disease
Epidemiology		
Prevalence in first-degree relatives	5%	10%
Concordance in monozygotic twins	10%	40%
Ethnic differences in prevalence	Yes	Yes
Disease associations (e.g. ankylosing spondylitis, Turner's syndrome)	Yes	Yes
Genetic abnormalities		
HLA-DR2	Increased (Japanese)	–
Susceptibility loci		
Chromosome 16q12 (*IBD1*, *CARD15 [NOD2]*)	–	Yes
Chromosome 5q31 (*IBD5*)	–	Yes
Chromosome 14q11 (*IBD4*)	–	Yes
Chromosome 6p13 (*IBD3*)	–	Yes
Chromosome 3p21	–	Yes
Chromosome 2	Yes	–
Chromosome 12q (*IBD2*)	Yes	–
Chromosomes 1, 3, 4, 7	Yes	Yes
Gene products and markers		
Increased gut permeability	Yes	Yes
Defective colonic mucus	Yes	–
Abnormal immune regulation	Yes	Yes
pANCA	Yes	–
ASCA	–	Yes

ASCA, anti-*Saccharomyces cerevisiae* antibody; HLA, human leukocyte antigen; pANCA, perinuclear antineutrophil cytoplasmic antibody.

IBD increases tenfold in the first-degree relatives of patients with ulcerative colitis, and the risk is even higher for relatives of patients with Crohn's disease. There is a high rate of concordance for IBD in monozygotic twins, again particularly in Crohn's disease (40% compared with 10% in ulcerative colitis).

Genetic studies. The results of genetic studies suggest that the two diseases are distinct, sharing some but not all susceptibility genes (Table 1.2). In particular, recent interest has focused on mutations in the caspase-activating recruitment domain gene, CARD15 (previously called NOD2), on chromosome 16 in patients with Crohn's disease.

IBD1, CARD15 (NOD2) gene. Two single-nucleotide polymorphisms and one frame-shift mutation of the CARD15 gene at the IBD1 locus on chromosome 16 have recently been reported to be associated with Crohn's disease. The risk of the disease is increased over fortyfold for individuals who are homozygous for all three polymorphisms. About 40% of European patients with familial Crohn's disease carry one of the three CARD15 mutations. Early reports indicate that CARD15 mutations predispose in particular to fibrostenosing small-bowel and right-sided colonic Crohn's disease.

The polymorphisms identified may confer susceptibility to Crohn's disease by altering monocyte recognition of the constituents of bacterial flora in the gut lumen and/or by modifying activation of the nuclear transcription factor NF-κB (nuclear factor κB). However, because CARD15 mutations account for only about 20–30% of cases and are not linked with Crohn's disease in Japanese patients, this genetic risk factor is neither necessary nor sufficient for the development of Crohn's disease. It seems likely that in the future other susceptibility genes that influence how the immune system interacts with the bacterial microenvironment within the gut will be identified.

Other gene products and genetic markers. It is not yet known how the other chromosomal susceptibility loci that have been identified so far might influence the pathogenesis and/or phenotype of IBD. It is likely, however, that some of the potentially pathophysiological abnormalities in IBD, such as increased gut permeability, defective colonic mucus and disordered immune regulation (Table 1.2), are genetically determined. For example, perinuclear antineutrophil cytoplasmic antibodies (pANCAs) are present in the serum of 50–80% of patients with ulcerative colitis (compared with only 5% of those with Crohn's disease); although not of pathogenetic importance, this presence is probably determined genetically. Definition of the genetic abnormalities underlying IBD is likely, in due course, to increase diagnostic accuracy and efficiency, to clarify and enable the prediction of disease phenotype, to facilitate family counseling, and to make it possible to forecast the therapeutic response in individual patients.

Environmental factors. Epidemiological and other evidence has identified a number of environmental factors that may play a role in the etiopathogenesis of IBD (Table 1.3).

Smoking. Only about 10% of patients with ulcerative colitis smoke, compared with 30% of the normal population and 40% of those with

TABLE 1.3

Environmental factors that may exacerbate inflammatory bowel disease

Factor	Ulcerative colitis	Crohn's disease
Cigarettes		
non-smoking	Yes	–
smoking	–	Yes
Dietary factors	Milk (rarely)	Various
Infection	Enteric infections	Under investigation
Drugs		
NSAIDs	Yes	Yes
antibiotics	Yes	Yes
oral contraceptives	Yes	Yes
Appendiceal inflammation	Yes	–
Stress	Yes	Yes

NSAIDs, non-steroidal anti-inflammatory drugs.

Crohn's disease. A history of recent cessation of smoking is common in patients presenting with ulcerative colitis for the first time, and nicotine patches have a modest therapeutic benefit. Conversely, in Crohn's disease smoking increases the risk of relapse and of surgery, while cessation improves the natural history of the disease. Nicotine and other constituents of tobacco smoke have a variety of effects on the inflammatory response, but it is not known why these are beneficial in patients with ulcerative colitis yet harmful in those with Crohn's disease.

Diet. In ulcerative colitis, up to 5% of patients improve by avoiding cows' milk, but no other potentially pathogenic dietary factors are known. Patients with active Crohn's disease improve when their ordinary food is replaced by a liquid formula diet, and they may deteriorate thereafter on the introduction of specific foods (see Chapter 6). However, no particular foods that are universally detrimental to patients with Crohn's disease have been identified.

Specific infection. Despite its resemblance to, and occasional onset after, infective diarrhea, there is no evidence that ulcerative colitis is due to a single infective agent. The possible roles of pathogenic *Escherichia coli* and sulfate-reducing bacteria are under investigation. Epidemiological, molecular biological and serological research has suggested initiating roles for *Mycobacterium paratuberculosis*, the measles virus and vaccination, and *Listeria monocytogenes* in the pathogenesis of Crohn's disease, but available data are controversial and require further evaluation.

Enteric microflora. Resident gut microflora are likely to be a major environmental factor in the pathogenesis of IBD. Circumstantial clinical and direct experimental evidence highlights the importance of the fecal stream in driving mucosal inflammation. The presence of gut flora is required for the full expression of enterocolitis in genetic and induced animal models of IBD. Patients with active IBD show loss of immunologic tolerance to intestinal microflora. Lastly, antibiotics and possibly probiotics have a therapeutic role in IBD.

Drugs. Relapse of IBD may be precipitated by nonsteroidal anti-inflammatory drugs (NSAIDs), perhaps as a result of inhibition of the synthesis of cytoprotective prostaglandins, and by antibiotics, probably secondary to changes in enteric flora. The oral contraceptive pill has been associated epidemiologically with Crohn's disease in particular: conceivably, the explanation is vascular (see below).

Appendectomy. Previous appendectomy is rare in patients developing ulcerative colitis: it has been suggested that T lymphocytes in an inflamed appendix could trigger inflammation (ulcerative colitis) in the more distal large bowel in genetically predisposed individuals.

Stress. Psychological stress is common in patients with IBD, particularly those with Crohn's disease, due to the unpleasant, chronic and intractable nature of their illness. It is possible, however, that in some patients, stress may itself trigger relapse of IBD, as has been shown in animal models, for example, by activation of leukocytes by enteric nerve endings in the gut wall (Figure 1.2).

Pathogenesis

The initiating factor(s) in IBD is (are) unknown, but we do know that altered immune regulation leads to a prolonged mucosal inflammatory response that is amplified and perpetuated by the recruitment of leukocytes from the gut vasculature. Upregulation of the expression of nuclear transcription factors, such as NF-κB, is likely to underlie the subsequent excessive local release of cytokines, growth factors, reactive oxygen metabolites, nitric oxide, eicosanoids (leukotrienes, thromboxanes, prostaglandins), platelet-activating factor, proteases, neuropeptides and other mediators (Figure 1.2). In ulcerative colitis, a non-T-helper lymphocyte (non-Th1) cytokine response generates a largely humoral immune profile, while in Crohn's disease, a cell-mediated response is induced by Th1s (Table 1.4).

Defective colonic mucus (in ulcerative colitis) and abnormal intestinal epithelial permeability (in both forms of IBD) may increase the access of luminal dietary and bacterial products to the mucosa. Impaired availability and metabolism of bacterially derived luminal short-chain fatty acids may adversely affect colonic epithelial function in ulcerative colitis, while in Crohn's disease, a procoagulant diathesis and multifocal granulomatous intestinal microinfarction may occur early in the disease process.

13

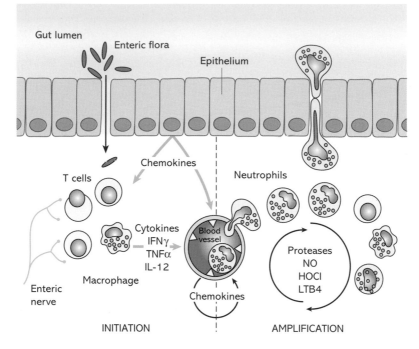

Figure 1.2 Mediators and mechanisms involved in the pathogenesis of IBD. The initiating factors are uncertain, but may include a breakdown in tolerance to enteric flora. T-cell and macrophage activation leads to production of cytokines, which act at several levels, including the local microvasculature, with generation of a chemokine gradient that causes transmigration of neutrophils, leading to tissue damage by metalloproteases and other reactive substances, augmentation of the inflammatory response and disruption of the epithelial barrier, itself causing further ingress of enteric flora and their products. The inflammatory response may be modulated by activation of lymphocytes by enteric nerve endings. HOCl, hypochlorite; IFNγ, interferon gamma; IL, interleukin; LTB4, leukotriene B4; NO, nitric oxide; TNFα, tumor necrosis factor α.

Lessons from animal models. Animal models, as indicated above, have provided valuable insights into the genetic, immune and environmental interactions involved in the etiopathogenesis of IBD. Gene knockout models, in particular, have shown that any of several different primary immune defects can lead to intestinal mucosal inflammation, as long as the animal has not been reared in germ-free conditions, thus confirming

TABLE 1.4

Immune and inflammatory response in inflammatory bowel disease

	Ulcerative colitis	Crohn's disease
Humoral immunity		
Association with auto-immune disease (Hashimoto's thyroiditis, SLE etc.)	Strong	Weak
Autoantibody production (anticolon antibody, pANCA etc.)	Common	Rare
Cell-mediated immunity		
Mucosal infiltrate	Non-granulomatous; neutrophils prominent	Granulomatous; T lymphocytes prominent
T-cell reactivity	Normal/decreased	Increased
Cytokine profile		
Th response	Non-Th1 (IL-10, IL-4, IL-13)	Th1 (IL-2, IFN, IL-12, TNFα)
Other cytokines	IL-1, IL-6, IL-8	IL-1, IL-6

IFN, interferon; IL, interleukin; SLE, systemic lupus erythematosus; Th, T-helper lymphocyte; TNFα, tumor necrosis factor α.

the central role of T cells and regulatory cytokines, and the importance of intestinal bacteria for full expression of the disease.

Pathology

The macroscopic and microscopic appearances of the bowel play a key role in the diagnosis of ulcerative colitis and Crohn's disease.

Ulcerative colitis. This usually begins in the rectum, and either remains there or spreads proximally (Figure 1.3). In severe total ulcerative colitis, the distal ileum ('backwash ileitis') is occasionally involved, but

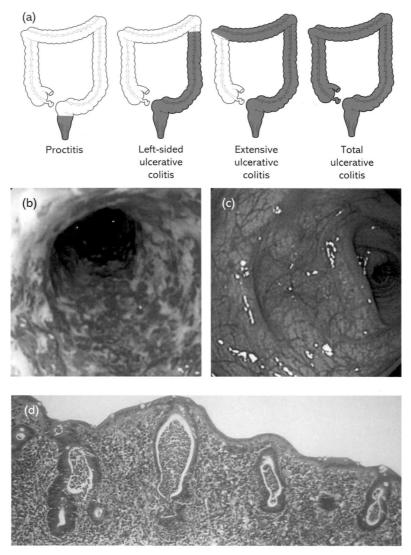

Figure 1.3 (a) Distribution of ulcerative colitis; (b) colonoscopic appearance of active ulcerative colitis – mucopurulent exudate, erythema, granularity and superficial ulceration; (c) normal colonic mucosa for comparison; (d) microscopic appearance of ulcerative colitis – intense inflammatory cell infiltration of the lamina propria, goblet-cell depletion and crypt abscesses. Photomicrograph courtesy of Dr RM Feakins, Barts and the London, Queen Mary School of Medicine and Dentistry, London, UK.

TABLE 1.5

Histology of inflammatory bowel disease

Feature	Ulcerative colitis	Crohn's disease
Lamina propria cell infiltrate	Diffuse, superficial; neutrophils prominent	Discontinuous, deep lymphocytes
Cryptitis, crypt abscesses	Prominent	Focal
Crypt distortion and loss	Widespread	Patchy
Goblet cell mucin depletion	Marked	Rare
Ulceration	Superficial	Deep
Epithelioid granulomas	None	Occasional

this is not clinically important. In the colon, there is diffuse mucosal inflammation with hyperemia, granularity, surface pus and blood, leading, in severe cases, to extensive ulceration. This heals by granulation to form multiple pseudopolyps.

Microscopically, acute and chronic inflammatory cells infiltrate the lamina propria and crypts (producing crypt abscesses). Crypt architecture is distorted and goblet cells lose their mucin (goblet cell depletion) (Table 1.5, Figure 1.3). The mucosa is edematous with epithelial ulceration. Biopsies in long-standing total colitis may show dysplasia, in which epithelial cell nuclei are enlarged and crowded, and lose their polarity: carcinoma may supervene (see below).

Crohn's disease. This can affect any part of the gut (Table 1.6). Typically, there are discontinuously affected gut segments (skip lesions). The first visible abnormality is lymphoid follicular enlargement with a surrounding ring of erythema (the 'red-ring' sign); this leads to aphthoid ulceration, which, in turn, progresses to deep fissuring ulcers with cobble-stoning, fibrosis, stricturing and fistulation (Figure 1.4). Inflammation and fibrosis predispose to intestinal strictures, presenting with obstructing symptoms, and to local perforation of the gut wall, leading to abscess formation (see below).

Histologically, there is transmural chronic inflammatory cell infiltration with ulceration and formation of micro-abscesses. Non-

17

TABLE 1.6

Sites of Crohn's disease

Site	Proportion of patients
Ileocecal	45%
Colitis only	25%
Terminal ileum only	20%
Extensive small bowel	5%
Other (anorectal, gastroduodenal, oral only)	5%

caseating epithelioid granulomas, sometimes containing multinucleate giant cells, are found in about 25% of patients investigated with colonoscopic biopsies, and in 60% of those examined after surgical resection of the bowel (Table 1.5, Figure 1.5). There is an increased risk of cancer in chronically inflamed areas of small intestinal, anorectal and particularly colorectal mucosa.

Indeterminate colitis. In some patients with chronic colitis, the pathological features are not typical of either ulcerative colitis or Crohn's disease. In these patients, the term 'indeterminate' colitis is used until or unless their colitis develops diagnostic characteristics.

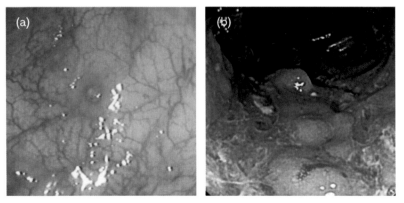

Figure 1.4 Colonoscopic appearances of Crohn's disease: (a) aphthous erosion in early disease; (b) ulceration and 'cobble-stoning' in well-established chronic disease.

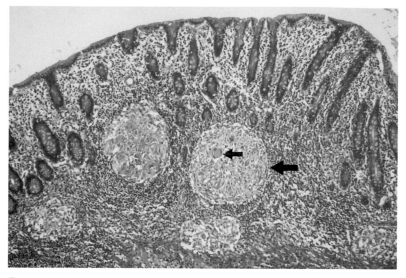

Figure 1.5 Microscopic appearance of colonic Crohn's disease. Three large epithelioid granulomas with multinucleate giant cells are visible; the large arrow shows a granuloma and the small arrow shows a giant cell. Photomicrograph courtesy of Dr RM Feakins, Barts and the London, Queen Mary School of Medicine and Dentistry, London, UK.

Key points – etiopathogenesis

- The incidence of Crohn's disease, but not that of ulcerative colitis, has risen steadily over recent decades.
- Clarification of the genetics of IBD is increasing our understanding of the etiopathogenesis of the disease. In the near future, it will also provide crucial information about phenotypic expression of the disease and the likely response of patients to therapy.
- Bacterial flora on the intestinal mucosa are likely to play a central role in driving mucosal inflammation in IBD.
- Smoking has contrasting effects in ulcerative colitis and Crohn's disease.
- The histology of affected gut mucosa provides essential clues to the diagnosis of IBD.

Key references

Bonen DK, Cho JH. The genetics of inflammatory bowel disease. *Gastroenterology* 2003;124:521–36.

Cope GF, Heatley RV. Cigarette smoking and intestinal defences. *Gut* 1992;33:721–3.

Cosnes J, Beaugerie L, Carbonnel F et al. Smoking cessation and the course of Crohn's disease: an intervention study. *Gastroenterology* 2001;120:1093–9.

Elson CO. Genes, microbes, and T-cells – new therapeutic targets in Crohn's disease. *N Engl J Med* 2002;346:614–16.

Fiocchi C. Inflammatory bowel disease: etiology and pathogenesis. *Gastroenterology* 1998;115: 182–205.

Hugot JP, Chamaillard M, Zouali H et al. Association of *NOD2* leucine-rich repeat variants with susceptibility to Crohn's disease. *Nature* 2001;411:599–603.

Ogura Y, Bonen DK, Inohara N et al. A frameshift mutation in *NOD2* associated with susceptibility to Crohn's disease. *Nature* 2001;411: 603–6.

Papadakis KA, Targan SR. Role of cytokines in the pathogenesis of inflammatory bowel disease. *Ann Rev Med* 2000;51:289–98.

Shanahan F. Inflammatory bowel disease: immunodiagnostics, immunotherapeutics, and ecotherapeutics. *Gastroenterology* 2001;120:622–35.

Clinical features of ulcerative colitis

The onset of ulcerative colitis is usually gradual, and its natural history chronic, with relapses and remissions over many years. Between attacks, patients are usually free of symptoms. Features of active disease depend on the extent as well as the activity of disease.

Acute severe ulcerative colitis most commonly occurs in patients with subtotal or total disease (see Figure 1.3) and causes profuse, frequent diarrhea (six or more loose stools per day) with blood and mucus, peridefecatory abdominal pain, fever, malaise, anorexia and weight loss. On external examination the patient is thin, anemic, fluid-depleted, febrile and tachycardic. In patients developing toxic megacolon and/or perforation, further deterioration is usually obvious, with sudden worsening of abdominal pain, distension, fever, tachycardia, sepsis and shock.

Moderate active ulcerative colitis is commonly left-sided (see Figure 1.3), causes rectal bleeding and discharge of mucus accompanied by diarrhea (less than six loose stools daily), urgency and sometimes abdominal pain. There may be malaise, but examination is usually normal.

Active proctitis causes rectal bleeding and mucous discharge, often with tenesmus and pruritus ani. There may be diarrhea, but the stool is often well-formed. Indeed, many patients with refractory proctitis (Chapter 5) are constipated. General health is usually maintained.

Clinical features of Crohn's disease

The symptoms and signs of Crohn's disease depend on its site and the predominant pathological process in each patient.

Active ileocecal and terminal ileal Crohn's disease usually present with pain and/or a tender mass in the right iliac fossa, with or without diarrhea and weight loss. Possible mechanisms of diarrhea include mucosal inflammation, bile-salt malabsorption (see Chapter 7) and bacterial overgrowth proximal to a stricture (Table 2.1). In patients with symptoms predominantly due to inflammation or abscess, the pain tends to be constant, often with fever. In patients with small-bowel obstruction, whether due to active inflammation or to fibrosis and stricture formation in the healing phase, the pain is more generalized, intermittent and colicky, and associated with loud borborygmi, abdominal distension, vomiting and eventually absolute constipation. Enterocutaneous fistulas are clinically obvious, but direct questions about pneumaturia and feculent vaginal discharge may be necessary to identify enterovesical or enterovaginal fistulas. Presentation as an acute abdomen, with peritonitis due to free perforation, is rare.

Active Crohn's colitis causes symptoms similar to those of active ulcerative colitis, although frank bleeding is less common. Extraintestinal manifestations (see below) are more common in Crohn's disease of the large than the small bowel.

TABLE 2.1

Mechanisms of diarrhea in Crohn's disease

Mechanism	Treatment
Inflammation	Anti-inflammatory drugs
Small-bowel bacterial overgrowth	Antibiotics
Bile-salt diarrhea	Colestyramine (cholestyramine)
Bile-salt deficiency	Low-fat diet
Lactase deficiency	Avoid lactose
Short bowel syndrome	See Table 2.2
Internal fistula	Surgery
Antibiotic-related	Stop antibiotics
Other (e.g. irritable bowel syndrome, celiac disease)	As appropriate

Extensive small-bowel Crohn's disease. As well as the above symptoms, patients with extensive small-bowel disease may have features of malabsorption, with steatorrhea, anemia and weight loss.

Perianal Crohn's disease is due to fissure, fistula (Figure 2.1) or abscess, and is suggested by perianal pain and/or discharge. It can be quickly confirmed in most patients by perineal inspection. Although perianal Crohn's disease is often much less uncomfortable than it looks, sigmoidoscopy (see Chapter 3) may be too painful to undertake without sedation or even anesthesia in some patients.

Gastroduodenal and oral Crohn's disease are both very rare. The former presents with upper abdominal pain or dyspepsia, often with anorexia, nausea, vomiting and weight loss, while the latter causes chronic oral ulceration and/or induration.

Intestinal complications of IBD

The main intestinal complications of IBD are undernutrition, short bowel syndrome and cancer.

Undernutrition. Nutritional deficiency is particularly common in Crohn's disease. Causes include reduced food intake, malabsorption in patients with small-bowel disease, increased loss of protein from an

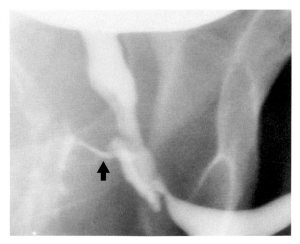

Figure 2.1

Micturating cystogram showing rectourethral fistula in Crohn's disease. The arrow indicates the fistula between the urethra and the rectum.

inflamed bowel, and increased metabolic requirements in sick patients, including the catabolic effects of cytokines and other inflammatory mediators. Patients at particular risk should be monitored carefully for evidence of undernutrition by measurement of weight, at least, and blood tests such as blood count, albumin, folate, vitamin B_{12} (cobalamin), ferritin, calcium and magnesium. Management options range from supplemental sip feeding with appropriate replacement of specific deficiencies, through enteral to parenteral nutrition (see Chapters 5 and 6).

Short bowel syndrome develops when extensive bowel resection leads to excessive malabsorption of fluids, electrolytes and nutrients. The most common cause is Crohn's disease, but it can also occur in patients with mesenteric vascular occlusion, trauma and neoplasia.

Pathogenesis. Factors influencing the symptoms experienced include the extent of resection(s), the presence of residual Crohn's disease and the absence of the ileocecal valve, which normally slows small-bowel transit and inhibits colonization of the distal small bowel by colonic flora. Furthermore, the site of resection is important: terminal ileal resection causes bile-salt malabsorption, vitamin B_{12} deficiency, gallstones and hyperoxaluria, while removal of the colon and small bowel causes severe diarrhea owing to loss of colonic absorptive capacity.

Presentation. Patients present with watery diarrhea immediately after resection. This tends to improve as the intestine adapts, or may progress to steatorrhea as bile-salt deficiency develops. Later complications include urinary stones and gallstones.

Investigation. Fluid, electrolyte and nutritional deficiencies, stool output, bile-salt malabsorption, vitamin B_{12} absorption and urinary oxalate excretion should be quantified.

Bile-salt malabsorption can be measured by means of SeHCAT scanning; SeHCAT (selenium-75-homocholic acid taurine) is a synthetic bile salt that emits gamma rays. After an oral dose, it is absorbed in the terminal ileum, and the amount retained after 7 days can be estimated by whole-body scanning. In patients with extensive ileal disease causing bile-salt malabsorption, retention is usually less than 15%.

Vitamin B_{12} absorption can be measured by the Schilling test. In the test, non-radioactive vitamin B_{12} is injected to saturate the body's stores; 2–6 hours later, radioactive vitamin B_{12} is ingested, with or without intrinsic factor. Urine is then collected over 24 hours to measure the absorption of vitamin B_{12}: reduced urinary excretion after oral administration of vitamin B_{12} with intrinsic factor indicates terminal ileal malabsorption of the vitamin.

Management. Intravenous restoration of fluid and electrolytes and total parenteral nutrition may be necessary at first. Enteral feeding is started early to promote gut adaptation using lactose-free iso-osmolar solutions (Table 2.2). Later, small, frequent meals are introduced, a low-fat diet being helpful for patients with marked steatorrhea. Excessive dietary oxalate should be avoided. Loperamide and codeine

TABLE 2.2

Management of short bowel syndrome

Supportive treatment

Intravenous fluids and nutrition initially

Enteral nutrition next

Small frequent low-fat meals later

Minimal dietary oxalate

Specific nutritional supplements as necessary
(calcium, magnesium, folate, vitamins, trace elements,
essential fatty acids)

Loperamide, codeine phosphate

Specific measures in severe cases

Calorie supplementation with medium-chain triglycerides

Gastric acid inhibition

Octreotide

Antibiotics for small-bowel overgrowth

Home total parenteral nutrition (refer to specialist center)

Small-bowel transplant (rarely)

phosphate may reduce stool output by slowing transit and increasing mucosal absorption.

In patients with extensive small-bowel resections, further treatment options include:
- dietary calorie supplements with medium-chain triglycerides (which are directly absorbed without having to be digested)
- H_2-receptor antagonists or proton-pump inhibitors (to reduce the gastric hypersecretion which can follow major gut resections)
- octreotide (to reduce gastric, biliary and pancreatic secretions)
- antibiotics (if there is small-bowel overgrowth).

Patients with massive resections who are unable to cope on exclusively oral nutrition need referral to specialist centers. They may need regular parenteral supplements of calcium, magnesium, trace elements, essential fatty acids and vitamins, or even total parenteral nutrition administered at home. Rarely, referral for small-bowel transplantation may be required.

Intestinal cancer

Colorectal carcinoma. Patients with chronic extensive ulcerative colitis have an increased risk of colorectal carcinoma, amounting to a cumulative risk of about 20% after 30 years of disease. Recent data indicate that patients with extensive Crohn's colitis are at similar risk. Factors increasing the risk of colorectal cancer in both diseases include chronicity of disease, coexistent primary sclerosing cholangitis (see below), family history of colorectal cancer, failure to use aminosalicylate drugs (see page 52) and folate deficiency. In both ulcerative colitis and Crohn's disease, most authorities advocate regular colonoscopic screening with multiple biopsies to detect epithelial dysplasia and/or early cancer, with a view to prompt surgical treatment. However, this approach has not yet been shown to reduce mortality from colorectal cancer in IBD.

Small intestinal and anal carcinoma. There is a small but finite risk of these otherwise rare cancers in patients with Crohn's disease: in particular, they occur at sites of very prolonged and severe inflammation.

Extraintestinal associations and complications of IBD

There are many systemic associations and complications of IBD; most affect the liver/biliary tree, joints, skin and eyes (Table 2.3). Most occur

TABLE 2.3

Extraintestinal associations and complications of inflammatory bowel disease

Organ	Complication
Joints/bones	Enteropathic arthropathy* Sacroiliitis Ankylosing spondylitis Clubbing (Crohn's disease only) Osteoporosis[†]
Eyes	Episcleritis* Uveitis*
Skin	Erythema nodosum* Pyoderma gangrenosum
Mouth	Aphthous ulceration
Liver	Fatty change Chronic active hepatitis Granulomatous hepatitis (Crohn's disease only) Cirrhosis Amyloid (Crohn's disease only)
Biliary tract	Cholesterol gallstones (terminal ileal Crohn's disease or resection)[†] Sclerosing cholangitis Cholangiocarcinoma
Kidneys	Uric acid stones (total colitis, ileostomy)[†] Oxalate stones (terminal ileal Crohn's disease or resection)[†]
Lungs	Fibrosing alveolitis
Blood	Anemia*[†] (iron, B_{12}, folate deficiency) Arterial and venous thrombosis[†]
Constitutional	Weight loss*[†] Growth retardation (children)*[†]

*Worse when IBD is active.
[†]Complication, rather than association.

in patients with colitis and some largely in those with active disease. In some instances, the condition appears to be a complication of IBD; for example, metabolic complications (gallstones and urinary stones). In others (ankylosing spondylitis, uveitis, arthropathy), there seems to be a genetic and/or immunologic association with IBD. In many cases, the pathogenesis is unknown. Extraintestinal associations and complications with important management implications are outlined below.

Sclerosing cholangitis occurs in about 5% of patients with ulcerative colitis and a smaller proportion of those with Crohn's disease. The pathogenesis is unknown, but it may occur years before the onset of overt colitis; 80% of patients have pANCAs in their serum. The condition is characterized by the gradual progression of an inflammatory obliterative fibrosis of the extra- and intrahepatic biliary tree (Figure 2.2), and is sometimes complicated by cholangiocarcinoma. The risk of colorectal cancer in patients with ulcerative colitis and sclerosing cholangitis excedes that associated with ulcerative colitis alone.

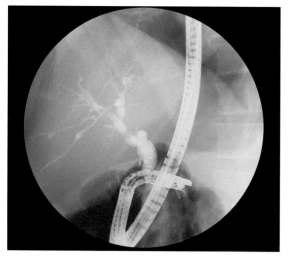

Figure 2.2 Primary sclerosing cholangitis on endoscopic retrograde cholangiopancreatography. Note how the multiple strictures, particularly in the intrahepatic biliary tree, give a beaded appearance.

Patients usually present with complications of biliary stricturing, such as obstructive jaundice, cholangitis or abnormal liver-function tests (raised alkaline phosphatase and gamma glutamyltranspeptidase) at routine screening. The diagnosis may be suggested by ultrasound, computed tomography (CT), magnetic resonance imaging (MRI) and/or liver biopsy; endoscopic retrograde cholangiopancreatography (ERCP) is useful not only for diagnosis (Figure 2.2), but also for the stenting of dominant strictures.

The course of sclerosing cholangitis is steadily progressive. Oral ursodeoxycholic acid improves pruritus and jaundice. Although it is of unproven benefit in relation to long-term outcome, ursodeoxycholic acid may reduce the incidence of colorectal cancer in patients with ulcerative colitis and sclerosing cholangitis. In patients not developing cholangiocarcinoma, liver transplant is the only hope of long-term survival; otherwise, median survival for symptomatic patients is about 15 years.

Joint disease

IBD-related arthropathy occurs in up to 10% of patients with IBD. The type of arthritis is determined by human leukocyte antigen (HLA) genotype. IBD-related arthropathy should not be confused with other musculoskeletal pains associated with IBD and its treatment; these include arthralgia related to steroid withdrawal, azathioprine-induced arthralgia and steroid-induced myopathy.

Pauciarticular disease involves fewer than five joints; characteristically, it affects one large joint, for example the knee, and is most common in women. Attacks usually coincide with relapse of colitis; sometimes there is simultaneous erythema nodosum or iritis. Its pathogenesis may involve deposition of gut-derived immune complexes in the affected joint in genetically predisposed individuals. Although the attacks of arthritis may come and go over many years, it is neither progressive nor deforming. In most patients, the joint symptoms resolve on treatment of the active ulcerative or Crohn's colitis with steroids or, if necessary, surgery. Sulfasalazine may be more effective for the joints than other aminosalicylates. Because aspirin and other NSAIDs may exacerbate IBD (see Chapter 1 under 'Environmental factors'), they should be avoided if possible. Alternatives include paracetamol and joint aspiration with steroid instillation.

Polyarticular IBD-related arthropathy affects more than five joints, particularly small joints such as the metacarpophalangeals. Symptoms are more common in women, are chronic and are not clearly related to activity of the associated IBD. Management resembles that of pauciarticular disease, except that response of the arthropathy to treatment of the IBD itself is poor.

Ankylosing spondylitis. While about 95% of patients without IBD who have ankylosing spondylitis are HLA-B27-positive, this is true of only 50–80% of patients with both diseases. Ankylosing spondylitis affects about 5% of patients with ulcerative or Crohn's colitis and, like enteropathic arthritis, is probably immunologically mediated. The patient presents with back pain and stiffness (Figure 2.3), diagnosis being confirmed by X-ray. There is often associated sacroiliitis. The course of ankylosing spondylitis is independent of the activity of IBD, and it may present years before the bowel disease becomes manifest. Treatment consists of vigorous physiotherapy, sulfasalazine and, if tolerated, NSAIDs (see above). Recent data indicate that infliximab (see 'Anti-TNFα antibodies' in Chapter 4) is an effective therapy in refractory ankylosing spondylitis.

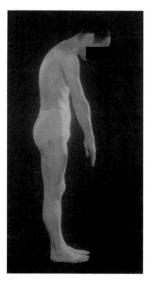

Figure 2.3 Ankylosing spondylitis, showing marked kyphosis. Reproduced courtesy of Dr DP D'Cruz, Guy's, King's and St Thomas' Hospital Medical School, London, UK.

Osteoporosis in IBD is a common consequence of chronic intestinal inflammation, malabsorption and treatment with corticosteroids, particularly a cumulative dose of more than 10 g prednisolone. Its exact prevalence is unclear. The disease is asymptomatic for many years, presenting eventually with vertebral collapse or long bone fractures. To prevent osteoporosis, all patients with IBD should be advised to eat a diet containing adequate calcium and vitamin D, supplemented if necessary by calcium and vitamin D tablets. They should avoid becoming either undernourished or obese (the latter not usually a problem in IBD), stop smoking and take regular exercise.

Patients at risk of osteoporosis should undergo bone densitometry. Those with established osteoporosis, or those needing long-term therapy with prednisolone, should receive cyclic bisphosphonate therapy (etidronate). The efficacy of oral budesonide (see Chapter 4) in preventing osteoporosis in steroid-dependent patients with Crohn's disease is not yet proven.

Hormone replacement therapy is associated with an increased risk of breast and gynecological cancer as well as of thromboembolic disease. Its use in the management of osteoporosis in postmenopausal women should be restricted to those in whom other treatments are ineffective or contraindicated.

Skin associations

Erythema nodosum occurs in about 8% of patients with ulcerative and Crohn's colitis, usually when the disease is active. Hot, red, tender nodules appear, usually on extensor surfaces of the lower legs and arms (Figure 2.4); they gradually subside after a few days to leave brownish skin discoloration. There may be an associated pauciarticular arthropathy. The diagnosis is clinical and biopsy is not necessary. Histology, if performed, shows vasculitis. Treatment is of the active associated IBD.

Pyoderma gangrenosum occurs during the course of IBD in about 2% of patients. There is no clear association with disease activity. Pyoderma presents initially as a discrete pustule with surrounding erythema; this develops into an indolent, painful enlarging ulcer. The most common site is the leg (Figure 2.5). Lesions are occasionally

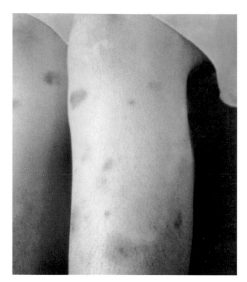

Figure 2.4
Erythema nodosum.

Figure 2.5
Pyoderma
gangrenosum:
(a) at presentation;
(b) in the healing
phase.

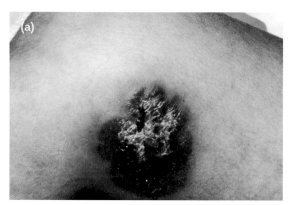

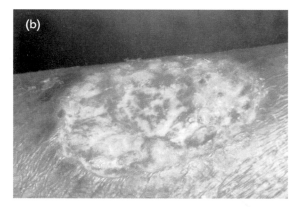

multiple and may occur at sites of recent trauma, for example operation scars. Histology shows lymphocytic vasculitis with dense secondary neutrophilic infiltration. Pyoderma is often refractory to treatment: options include intralesional, topical and systemic corticosteroids, dapsone, heparin, immunosuppressive drugs such as ciclosporin, and infliximab. Colectomy does not reliably induce healing of the skin lesion.

Ocular associations. The most common ocular associations of IBD are episcleritis and uveitis. Together they occur in less than 5% of patients, usually when the bowel disease is active. Episcleritis presents with burning and itching accompanied by a localized area of dilated blood vessels at the site of scleral inflammation (Figure 2.6). Topical steroids and treatment of the active IBD usually produce a satisfactory response. Uveitis is a more serious and often recurrent problem, presenting with headache, red eye and blurred vision; slit-lamp examination shows pus in the anterior chamber. Treatment includes topical steroids, cycloplegics and therapy of the active IBD. All patients with IBD complicated by ocular symptoms should be promptly referred to an ophthalmologist.

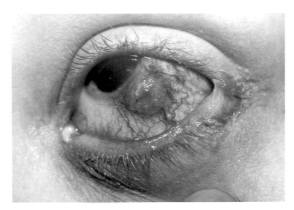

Figure 2.6 Episcleritis in a patient with active ulcerative colitis.

Key points – clinical features and complications

- The presentation of ulcerative colitis depends on its activity and extent, while that of Crohn's disease depends also on the underlying pathological process.
- Intestinal complications of IBD include undernutrition, short bowel syndrome (in Crohn's disease only) and cancer, particularly of the colon.
- The skin, joint, ocular and hepatic associations of IBD are most common in patients with colonic disease.
- The course of sclerosing cholangitis and ankylosing spondylitis is unrelated to the activity of the associated IBD.

Key references

Anonymous. AGA technical review on short bowel syndrome and intestinal transplantation. *Gastroenterology* 2003;124: 1111–34.

Bernstein CN, Blanchard JF, Kliewer E et al. Cancer risk in patients with inflammatory bowel disease: a population-based study. *Cancer* 2001;91:854–62.

Bernstein CN, Blanchard JF, Rawsthorne P et al. The prevalence of extraintestinal diseases in inflammatory bowel disease: a population-based study. *Am J Gastroenterol* 2001;96:1116–22.

Han PD, Burke A, Baldassano RN et al. Nutrition and inflammatory bowel disease. *Gastroenterol Clin N Am* 1999;28:423–43.

Lindor KD. Ursodiol for primary sclerosing cholangitis. Mayo Primary Sclerosing Cholangitis– Ursodeoxycholic Acid Study Group. *N Engl J Med* 1997;336:691–5.

Orchard TR, Thiyagaraja S, Welsh KI et al. Clinical phenotype is related to HLA genotype in the peripheral arthropathies of inflammatory bowel disease. *Gastroenterology* 2000; 118:274–8.

Orchard TR, Wordsworth BP, Jewell DP. Peripheral arthropathies in inflammatory bowel disease: their articular distribution and natural history. *Gut* 1998;42:387–91.

Rasmussen HH, Fallingborg JF, Mortensen PB et al. Hepatobiliary dysfunction and primary sclerosing cholangitis in patients with Crohn's disease. *Scand J Gastroenterol* 1997; 32:604–10.

Soukiasian S, Foster CS, Raizman MB. Treatment strategies for scleritis and uveitis associated with inflammatory bowel disease. *Am J Ophthalmol* 1994;118:601–11.

Tung BY, Emond MJ, Haggitt RC et al. Ursodiol use is associated with lower prevalence of colonic neoplasia in patients with ulcerative colitis and primary sclerosing cholangitis. *Ann Intern Med* 2001;134:89–95.

Differential diagnosis

The differential diagnosis of common presentations of IBD is shown in Tables 3.1–3.4. In younger patients (under 50 years) the main differential diagnoses, depending on presentation, include infection and irritable bowel syndrome. In older people (over 50 years), neoplasia, diverticular disease and ischemia require special consideration.

TABLE 3.1

Causes of bloody diarrhea

Cause	Disease
Inflammatory	Ulcerative colitis
	Crohn's colitis
	Behçet's colitis
Infective colitis	*Campylobacter*
	Salmonella
	Shigella
	Clostridium difficile
	Yersinia
	Tuberculosis
	Enterohemorrhagic *Escherichia coli* (VTEC/0157:H7)
	Amebiasis
	Schistosomiasis
	Cytomegalovirus*
	Herpes simplex*
Neoplastic	Colorectal cancer
Vascular	Ischemia
Iatrogenic	NSAIDs
	Antibiotics
	Irradiation

*Particularly in immunocompromised patients.
NSAIDs, non-steroidal anti-inflammatory drugs.

TABLE 3.2

Causes of rectal bleeding

Cause	Disease
Inflammatory	Proctitis
	Crohn's disease
Sexually transmitted	Gonococcus
	Cytomegalovirus
	Herpes simplex
	Atypical mycobacterium
	Chlamydia
	Kaposi's sarcoma
Neoplasia	Colorectal polyps
	Colorectal cancer
	Anal cancer
Vascular	Ischemia
	Angiodysplasia
Iatrogenic	NSAIDs (oral or suppositories)
	Irradiation
Other	Benign solitary rectal ulcer
	Diverticulosis (acute bleeds only)
	Severe upper gastrointestinal bleeding

NSAIDs, non-steroidal anti-inflammatory drugs.

Investigation

The aims of investigation (Tables 3.5 and 3.6) are to establish the diagnosis, its site, extent and activity, and to check for complications of the disease and its treatment.

Blood tests

Hematology. In patients presenting with abdominal pain and/or diarrhea, test results revealing anemia, raised platelet count and raised erythrocyte sedimentation rate (ESR) may suggest active IBD, but are not diagnostic. Patients with extensive chronic terminal ileal Crohn's disease may have low serum B_{12}, while a low red-cell folate may indicate active chronic inflammation, reduced intake or malabsorption.

TABLE 3.3

Causes of abdominal pain, diarrhea and weight loss

Cause	Disease
Inflammatory	Crohn's disease
	Ulcerative colitis
	Microscopic/lymphocytic/collagenous colitis*
	Behçet's colitis
Infections	See Table 3.1
Neoplasia	Colorectal cancer
	Pancreatic cancer
	Small-bowel lymphoma
	Endocrine tumors (carcinoid, gastrinoma, VIPoma)
Endocrine	Thyrotoxicosis
	Diabetic autonomic neuropathy
	Hypoadrenalism
Vascular	Ischemia
Iatrogenic	NSAIDs
	Antibiotics
	Laxative abuse
	Irradiation
	Gut resections
Malabsorption	Celiac disease
	Bacterial overgrowth
	Lactose intolerance†
Other	Irritable bowel syndrome†

*Pain and weight loss unusual.
†Weight loss unusual.
VIP, vasoactive intestinal polypeptide.

Iron deficiency is common, although again it is not diagnostic of IBD.

Regular blood counts are necessary to check for bone-marrow depression in patients maintained on immunosuppressive drugs such as azathioprine. Patients receiving sulfasalazine are at risk of hemolytic anemia and folate deficiency as well as bone-marrow depression.

Biochemistry. Raised C-reactive protein and low serum albumin levels suggest active disease in patients with established ulcerative

TABLE 3.4

Causes of abdominal pain and mass in the right iliac fossa

Cause	Disease
Ileocecal	
Inflammatory	Crohn's disease
	Appendiceal mass
Infective	Tuberculosis
	Ameboma
	Actinomycosis
Neoplastic	Cecal carcinoma
	Lymphoma
	Carcinoid tumor
Other	Fecal loading
Renal	Hydronephrosis
	Cysts
	Neoplasia
	Transplant
Gynecological	Ovarian cyst
	Neoplasia
	Tubal mass, including ectopic pregnancy
	Endometriosis

colitis or Crohn's disease; they are also suggestive, although not diagnostic, of IBD in those in whom the diagnosis has not yet been made. Low serum albumin, calcium, magnesium, zinc and essential fatty acid concentrations may be found in Crohn's disease patients with malabsorption, while abnormal liver-function tests may be found in patients with hepatobiliary complications of IBD, and require regular monitoring in patients on immunosuppressive therapy.

Serology. In patients presenting for the first time with diarrhea, a negative test for endomysial or transglutaminase antibodies usually excludes celiac disease as the diagnosis. Most patients with ulcerative colitis and a minority with Crohn's disease have circulating pANCAs, but this test is not sufficiently sensitive or specific to be of diagnostic value. The diagnostic usefulness of detection of circulating antibodies

39

TABLE 3.5

Laboratory investigation of inflammatory bowel disease

Sample	Test
Blood	
Hematology	Hemoglobin
	White blood cells
	Platelets
	Erythrocyte sedimentation rate
	Ferritin
	Vitamin B_{12} (Crohn's disease)
	Red-cell folate
Biochemistry	C-reactive protein
	Liver-function tests
	Albumin
	Calcium, magnesium (suspected malabsorption)
Serology	Endomysial or transglutaminase antibody*
(selected patients)	Amebiasis
	Strongyloidiasis
	Schistosomiasis
	HIV
Stools	Microscopy
	Culture
	Clostridium difficile toxin
	Calprotectin

*To exclude celiac disease.

to *Saccharomyces cerevisiae* (ASCA), which are present in most patients with small intestinal Crohn's disease, is also unclear. Conceivably, assays for both of these antibodies may prove useful in the future in patients with indeterminate disease.

For patients who have recently traveled to endemic areas, serology (as well as stool samples; see below) should be checked for amebiasis, strongyloidiasis and schistosomiasis. The use of corticosteroids in such patients, in the mistaken belief that they have active IBD, can have fatal consequences. HIV testing should be considered in patients at risk who have severe diarrhea.

TABLE 3.6

Endoscopy, histopathology and imaging for inflammatory bowel disease

Modality	Test
Endoscopy with biopsy	Sigmoidoscopy (outpatient department)
	Colonoscopy
	Gastroscopy (Crohn's disease, rarely)
	Enteroscopy (Crohn's disease, rarely)
	Wireless capsule endoscopy (Crohn's disease, rarely)
Conventional radiology	Chest X-ray (selected patients)
	Abdominal X-ray
	Barium follow-through or small-bowel enema (Crohn's disease only)
	Fistulography (rarely)
	Barium enema (rarely)
Isotope scanning	^{99}Tc-HMPAO-labeled leukocyte scan
Other imaging (mainly for Crohn's disease)	Ultrasound (transabdominal and endoscopic)
	CT scan
	MRI

CT, computed tomography; MRI, magnetic resonance imaging; ^{99}Tc-HMPAO, ^{99}technetium hexamethyleneamine oxime.

Stool tests

Microscopy. Fresh stools often show red and white blood cells in patients with active colitis, whether due to IBD or infection. Hot fresh samples are essential in recent travellers to look for amebic trophozoites.

Culture and toxin assay. Whether or not a diagnosis of IBD has already been made, patients presenting with diarrhea should always have stool samples sent for culture and to check for *Clostridium difficile* toxin. Patients with known ulcerative colitis occasionally present in relapse as a result of intercurrent infection, and require appropriate antibiotic therapy.

Fecal calprotectin. The transmigration of neutrophils through the mucosa into the lumen is responsible for crypt abscesses and exudate formation. This phenomenon has been exploited to devise an improved marker of disease activity, particularly in Crohn's disease. Fecal levels of calprotectin, a neutrophil-derived cytosolic protein that is resistant to bacterial degradation, provide an accurate index of intestinal inflammatory activity. Although not yet routinely available, the test is uncomplicated and promises to be a useful adjunct to routine outpatient clinical assessment.

Sigmoidoscopy and rectal biopsy

Ulcerative colitis. In patients presenting with diarrhea with or without rectal bleeding, rigid or flexible sigmoidoscopy in the unprepared patient, and without excessive air insufflation, can provide immediate confirmation of colitis and its activity (Figure 3.1). Sigmoidoscopy also allows biopsy for histology. To minimize the risks of bleeding and perforation, a small superficial biopsy should be taken from the posterior rectal wall less than 100 mm from the anal margin using small-cupped forceps. In patients with established ulcerative colitis, rectal biopsy is not routinely necessary. However, in those presenting for the first time, infective colitis as opposed to chronic ulcerative colitis may be suggested by histology showing an acute, focal and superficial infiltrate with minimal goblet-cell depletion and preservation of crypt architecture. Colitis due to C. *difficile*, cytomegalovirus, amebiasis or Crohn's disease often has a characteristic macroscopic appearance, but histology can be used to confirm these diagnoses.

Crohn's disease. Rectal sparing is common in Crohn's colitis. Sometimes, however, rectal induration or ulceration, or the presence of perianal disease, points to the diagnosis. Furthermore, in a minority of patients with macroscopically normal rectal mucosa but who have Crohn's disease proximal to this site, histology of rectal biopsies shows epithelioid granulomas (see Figure 1.5).

Colonoscopy and biopsy

Ulcerative colitis. In patients who are not severely ill, colonoscopy is the most useful test for confirming the diagnosis of ulcerative colitis

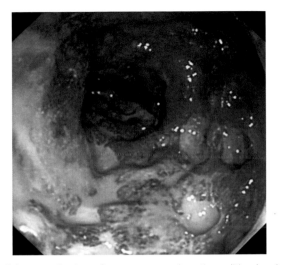

Figure 3.1 Colonoscopic view of acute severe ulcerative colitis, showing deep ulcers with epithelial denudation adjacent to erythematous, edematous mucosa.

and assessing disease extent and activity. It has the advantage over barium enema and radiolabeled leukocyte scanning (see below) of allowing biopsies to be taken. Macroscopically, inactive ulcerative colitis is characterized by mucosal edema with loss of the normal vascular pattern, erythema and granularity, while in patients with active disease, there is, additionally, contact or spontaneous bleeding, excessive mucopus and surface ulceration (Figure 3.1). In chronic cases, pseudopolyps and loss of the normal haustral pattern with apparent shortening of the colon are common, and in very long-standing disease, the mucosa becomes atrophic.

In patients with acute severe ulcerative colitis, colonoscopy may cause perforation and dilation, and most sick patients can be managed satisfactorily without it. However, colonoscopy plays a major role in cancer surveillance in patients with chronic extensive ulcerative colitis (see page 89).

Crohn's disease. Colonoscopy with terminal ileoscopy is central to the macroscopic and microscopic diagnosis of Crohn's disease. It can also be used to balloon-dilate short strictures. In early Crohn's disease, prominent lymphoid follicles (the red-ring sign) are followed by aphthoid ulceration. Later, larger pleomorphic deep ulcers develop, separated by relatively normal-looking mucosa. A cobble-stone appearance of the mucosa is a late sign (see Figure 1.4b). Changes in the colon are often segmentally distributed (skip lesions).

Wireless capsule endoscopy. The recent advent of wireless capsule endoscopy enables non-invasive visualization of small bowel that is inaccessible to the conventional endoscope. Use of this test for the diagnosis of Crohn's disease, however, may be compromised by the inability of the capsule, at present, to take biopsies (see below). Furthermore, patients with intestinal strictures are at risk of capsule-induced obstruction.

Radiology
Plain abdominal X-ray
Ulcerative colitis. In patients presenting with active disease, a plain film is useful to assess the extent of disease, since fecal residue on X-ray usually indicates sites of uninflamed colonic mucosa. Plain abdominal radiography is also used to exclude colonic dilation (diameter more than 55 mm) in patients with acute severe ulcerative colitis (Figure 3.2).

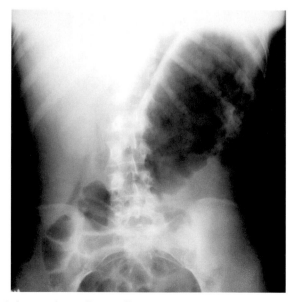

Figure 3.2 Acute colonic dilation affecting the transverse colon.

In this setting, severe disease is also indicated by deep ulceration and coarse nodularity of the mucosa, or 'mucosal islands', and linear gas-tracking in the gut wall.

Crohn's disease. A plain film (preferably both supine and erect) is essential if small-bowel obstruction is suspected. It may also hint at a mass in the right iliac fossa, and is helpful, as in ulcerative colitis, in estimating disease extent or severity in active Crohn's colitis. Classically, but exceptionally, complicating radio opaque urinary stones or gallstones are seen (Table 2.3; see also Chapter 7).

Contrast and air enemas. Conventional double-contrast barium enema (Figure 3.3) has largely been superseded by colonoscopy (see above). In patients with active colitis, 'air enemas', in which air is gently introduced into the unprepared rectum, are performed in some centers to enhance the information provided by plain abdominal X-ray; in others, 'instant' barium enema is performed without bowel preparation. Neither technique, however, adds materially to management in most patients, and both carry a small risk of causing colonic perforation or dilation in severely ill individuals.

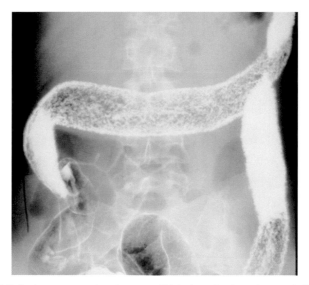

Figure 3.3 Barium enema showing superficial ulceration in active total ulcerative colitis. This test has now been largely superseded by colonoscopy in patients with ulcerative colitis; both tests are potentially dangerous in active disease.

Small-bowel radiology. Contrast examination of the small bowel is of central importance in the diagnosis of Crohn's disease proximal to the terminal ileum, showing strictures, ulceration and fistulation (Figure 3.4). Arguments persist about whether conventional barium follow-through or small-bowel enema (enteroclysis) is preferable, but both should be avoided in severely ill patients with Crohn's disease.

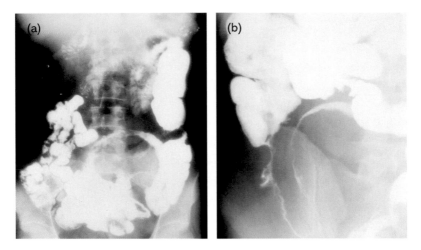

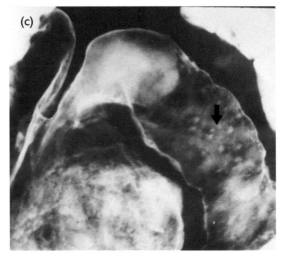

Figure 3.4 Radiological appearance of the small bowel in 3 patients with Crohn's disease: (a) skip lesions causing stricturing at several sites in ileum; (b) single long terminal ileal stricture; (c) aphthous ulcers (arrowed) in terminal ileum.

Enteroclysis may be more sensitive than barium follow-through for the diagnosis of small lesions and short strictures, but many patients find the necessary duodenal intubation very uncomfortable. Contrast fistulography is a useful way of clarifying anatomic connections in patients with abdominal sinuses or fistulas.

Radiolabeled leukocyte scans. The intensity and extent of colonic uptake 1 hour after injection of autologous, radiolabeled leukocytes provides information, non-invasively, about disease activity, particularly the extent and site, where doubt exists in patients with ulcerative colitis or Crohn's disease (Figure 3.5). Labeling with ^{99}Tc-hexamethylene-amine oxime (^{99}Tc-HMPAO) is preferable to ^{111}indium because of its superior definition, lower radiation dose, shorter scanning interval and lower cost. Increased isotopic activity on such scans is not, of course, specific for IBD, since positive results are obtained in other inflammatory gut diseases.

Delayed scanning can be very helpful in identifying an intra-abdominal abscess, for example in patients with Crohn's disease. In patients with mucosal inflammation, delayed scans outline more distal bowel as the radiolabeled leukocytes that have migrated into the lumen move distally. In patients with an abscess, however, the site of uptake remains constant, often gradually intensifying.

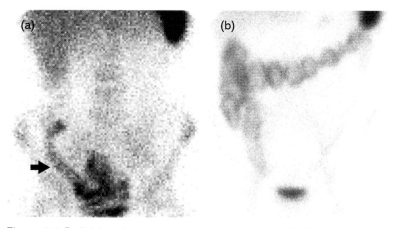

Figure 3.5 Radiolabeled leukocyte scans in two patients with Crohn's disease showing inflammation in: (a) the distal ileum (arrowed); (b) the terminal ileum, cecum and ascending and transverse colon.

Ultrasound, CT scanning and MRI. In active Crohn's disease, but not ulcerative colitis, abdominal ultrasound and CT scanning can be very useful, allowing not only the evaluation but also the percutaneous drainage of localized collections. Computed tomography will precisely define the anatomy of fistulas and sinuses in Crohn's disease, while both techniques are also increasingly used for identifying intrinsic gut-wall abnormalities, such as areas of thickening or matting of bowel loops. Endoluminal ultrasound and MRI provide the most accurate delineation of perianal abscesses and fistulas.

Key points – diagnosis

- The aims of investigation are to diagnose IBD, distinguish between ulcerative colitis and Crohn's disease, establish its site, extent and activity, and check for complications of the disease and its treatment.
- Laboratory, endoscopic, histological and imaging tests should be regarded as complementary, but should be undertaken selectively according to the presentation of individual patients.

Key references

Bartram CI. Radiology in the current assessment of ulcerative colitis. *Gastrointest Radiol* 1977;25:383–92.

Gaya DR, Mackenzie JF. Faecal calprotectin: a bright future for assessing disease activity in Crohn's disease. *QJM* 2002;95:557–8.

Giaffer MH. Labelled leucocyte scintigraphy in inflammatory bowel disease: clinical applications. *Gut* 1996;38:1–5.

Iddan G, Meron G, Glukhovsky A et al. Wireless capsule endoscopy. *Nature* 2000;405:417.

Parente F, Maconi G, Bollani S et al. Bowel ultrasound in assessment of Crohn's disease and detection of related small bowel strictures: a prospective comparative study versus x-ray and intraoperative findings. *Gut* 2002;50:490–5.

Scholmerich J. Inflammatory bowel disease. *Endoscopy* 2003;35:164–70.

Wills JS, Lobis IF, Denstman FJ. Crohn's disease: state of the art. *Radiology* 1997;202:597–610.

This chapter outlines the pharmacology, mechanism of action, indications, side effects, monitoring and contraindications of drugs currently used as specific anti-inflammatory agents in ulcerative colitis and Crohn's disease. Imminent and future developments in medical therapy are also considered.

Corticosteroids

The corticosteroids used in IBD, their indications and their side effects are listed in Table 4.1.

Pharmacology. Corticosteroids can be given intravenously, orally or topically (as a suppository or an enema), the route selected depending on the severity and site of disease. The most widely used oral preparation is prednisolone. Intravenous alternatives are hydrocortisone and methylprednisolone. The former may be marginally more effective in acute severe ulcerative colitis, but it has a greater mineralocorticoid effect. Adrenocorticotropic hormone injections are no longer used: although they are efficacious in patients with acute severe ulcerative colitis who have not previously used oral steroids, they offer no practical advantages over conventional corticosteroids.

The systemic side effects of conventional steroids (Table 4.1) have prompted a search for safer formulations. For topical therapy of distal ulcerative colitis, several enema preparations containing steroids that are poorly absorbed and/or undergo rapid first-pass intestinal mucosal and hepatic metabolism are available (e.g. prednisolone metasulfo-benzoate and budesonide). These preparations produce fewer systemic side effects and less adrenocortical suppression than hydrocortisone and prednisolone sodium phosphate enemas. A more important advance is the introduction of an oral, controlled ileal-release formulation of budesonide for the treatment of active ileocecal Crohn's disease. This drug resembles oral prednisolone in efficacy, but, because of its rapid first-pass metabolism, causes much less adrenocortical suppression, as

TABLE 4.1

Corticosteroids in inflammatory bowel disease

Preparations

Intravenous	Hydrocortisone (300–400 mg/day)
	Methylprednisolone (40–60 mg/day)
Oral	Prednisolone, prednisolone enteric-coated,
	prednisone (up to 60 mg/day)
	Budesonide (up to 9 mg/day)
Enemas	Liquid: prednisolone metasulfobenzoate,
	prednisolone sodium phosphate, budesonide
	Foam: prednisolone metasulfobenzoate
	(Predfoam), hydrocortisone (Colifoam)
Suppositories	Hydrocortisone, prednisolone sodium
	phosphate (Predsol)

Indications   Active ulcerative colitis and Crohn's disease

Side effects

General	Cushingoid facies, weight gain, dysphoria
Metabolic	Adrenocortical suppression, hyperglycemia,
	hypokalemia
Cardiovascular	Hypertension, fluid retention
Infection	Opportunistic infections, reactivation of
	tuberculosis, severe chickenpox
Skin	Acne, bruising, striae, hirsuties
Eyes	Cataracts, glaucoma
Musculoskeletal	Osteoporosis, avascular osteonecrosis, myopathy
Children	Growth retardation

Monitoring   Blood pressure, blood sugar/potassium

Contraindications Poorly controlled diabetes or hypertension
(all relative)   Osteoporosis
              Active peptic ulcer
              Concurrent serious infections

(CONTINUED)

TABLE 4.1 (CONTINUED)

Mechanisms of action

Leukocytes	Reduced migration, activation, survival
	Reduced activation of NF-κB
	Phospholipase A2 inhibition
	Reduced induction of Cox-2 and inducible NOS
	Reduced production of cytokines and lipid mediators
	Increased kinin degradation
Endothelial cells	Reduced expression of adhesion molecules
	Reduced capillary permeability

Cox, cyclo-oxygenase; NF-κB, nuclear transcription factor κB; NOS, nitric oxide synthase.

assessed by plasma cortisol levels. However, it is more expensive than prednisolone. Controlled colonic-release formulations of budesonide and of prednisolone for use in ulcerative and Crohn's colitis are under evaluation.

Mechanism of action. By combining with intracellular glucocorticoid receptors, corticosteroids have many potentially beneficial actions on the inflammatory process (Table 4.1; see also Chapter 1), but which of these is, or are, of predominant importance in IBD is unclear.

Indications. The use of corticosteroids should be restricted to the treatment of patients with active ulcerative colitis and Crohn's disease, as there is no evidence that they are able to maintain remission. Further details are given in Chapters 5 and 6.

Side effects. The principal side effects of corticosteroids are listed in Table 4.1. They are related to both dose and duration, except for avascular osteonecrosis, which is unpredictable and may occur after only short courses of treatment.

Monitoring treatment. The small minority of patients with IBD who require long-term treatment with oral corticosteroids should have regular checks of their blood pressure and blood sugar and potassium concentrations. Patients who exceed a cumulative dose of about 10 g of prednisolone should be assessed for osteoporosis by bone densitometry and treated accordingly (see Chapter 2).

Contraindications. In patients with poorly controlled diabetes mellitus or hypertension, and in those with established osteoporosis or peptic ulceration, alternative pharmacological treatments should be used when possible. If steroid therapy is unavoidable, topical therapy or oral budesonide (in patients with ileocecal Crohn's disease) is preferable to oral prednisolone.

Aminosalicylates

Pharmacology. 5-Aminosalicylates (5-ASAs) are available in oral formulations (Table 4.2) and as enemas and suppositories (Table 4.3). The original compound, sulfasalazine, consists of 5-aminosalicylic acid linked by an azo bond to sulfapyridine (Figure 4.1; Table 4.2). The sulfonamide moiety acts as a carrier to deliver 5-ASA, the active component, to the colon, where it is released by bacterial action. About 20% of patients cannot tolerate sulfasalazine because of side effects, most of which are due to sulfapyridine (Table 4.3).

The newer oral 5-ASA formulations (Table 4.2) are much better tolerated than sulfasalazine (see below). The pH-dependent, delayed-release and, particularly, slow-release mesalazine preparations also release 5-ASA more proximally in the gut, making them potentially useful in small-bowel Crohn's disease as well as in ulcerative and Crohn's colitis (Figure 4.2). In contrast, olsalazine and balsalazide, like sulfasalazine, release 5-ASA by bacterial azo reduction in the colon and are indicated for use only in colitis. Because of their greater tolerability and safety, it is hard to justify not prescribing one of the newer derivatives to a patient presenting for the first time with IBD. However, in the absence of side effects, patients who are already well established on sulfasalazine need not be switched to an alternative formulation.

Mechanism of action. Like corticosteroids, aminosalicylates have a wide variety of anti-inflammatory effects (Table 4.3). However, it is not known which of these explains their efficacy in IBD.

TABLE 4.2

Representative examples of oral formulations of aminosalicylates (5-ASAs) in inflammatory bowel disease

Drug	Formulation	Dose range (maintenance– conventional maximum)
Prodrugs (5-ASA azo-linked to carrier)		
Sulfasalazine	5-ASA–sulfapyridine	1 g twice daily – 2 g three times daily
Olsalazine	5-ASA–5-ASA	500 mg twice daily – 1 g three times daily
Balsalazide	5-ASA–aminobenzoylalanine	1.5 g twice daily – 2.25 g three times daily
Mesalazine (5-ASA alone)		
Delayed-release		
Asacol	Eudragit S coating dissolves at pH > 7	400–800 mg three times daily
Salofalk	Eudragit L coating dissolves at pH > 6	500 mg – 1 g three times daily
Slow-release		
Pentasa	Ethylcellulose microspheres	500 mg three times daily – 2 g twice daily
Salofalk	Granules	500 mg – 1 g three times daily

Sites to which 5-ASAs are delivered from these formulations are shown in Figure 4.2.

Indications and choice of preparation. 5-ASA compounds have a therapeutic role in moderately active (although not acute severe) ulcerative colitis and, particularly, in the prevention of relapse in patients with inactive disease. Taken long-term, 5-ASA drugs may reduce the risk of development of colorectal cancer in patients with extensive ulcerative colitis. In patients with left-sided ulcerative colitis, drugs delivering 5-ASA primarily to the colon (olsalazine, balsalazide)

53

TABLE 4.3

Aminosalicylates in inflammatory bowel disease

Preparations

Oral	See Table 4.2
Enemas	Liquid: Pentasa, Salofalk, sulfasalazine Foam: Asacolfoam, Salofalk foam
Suppositories	Asacol, Pentasa, Salofalk, sulfasalazine

Indications Active and inactive ulcerative colitis
Active and inactive Crohn's disease (possibly;
   see Chapter 6)

Side effects

General	Headache,* fever*
Gut	Nausea,* vomiting,* diarrhea, exacerbation of ulcerative colitis

Blood	Hemolysis,* folate deficiency,* agranulocytosis,*
	   thrombocytopenia,* aplastic anemia,*
	   methemoglobinemia*

Renal	Orange urine,* interstitial nephritis
Skin	Rashes,* toxic epidermal necrolysis,* Stevens–Johnson syndrome,* hair loss
Other	Oligospermia,* acute pancreatitis, hepatitis, lupus syndrome, myocarditis, pulmonary fibrosis

Monitoring

Sulfasalazine	Every 3 months: blood count, red-cell folate, serum urea/creatinine, liver-function tests
Mesalazine	Every 6–12 months: serum urea/creatinine

Contraindications

Sulfasalazine	Known salicylate or sulfonamide sensitivity, G6PDH deficiency, porphyria
Mesalazine	Salicylate sensitivity, renal failure

(CONTINUED)

TABLE 4.3 (CONTINUED)

Mechanisms of action

Leukocytes
Reduced migration, cytotoxicity
Reduced activation of NF-κB
Reduced synthesis of IL-1 and lipid mediators
Reduced degradation of prostaglandins
Antioxidant
TNF antagonist
Reduced fMLP receptor binding

Epithelium
Reduced MHC Class II expression
Induction of heat shock proteins
Reduced apoptosis

*Side effects usually due to sulfonamide component of sulfasalazine.

fMLP, formyl–methionyl–leucyl–phenylalanine; G6PDH, glucose-6-phosphate dehydrogenase; IL, interleukin; MHC, major histocompatibility complex; NF-κB, nuclear transcription factor κB; TNF, tumor necrosis factor.

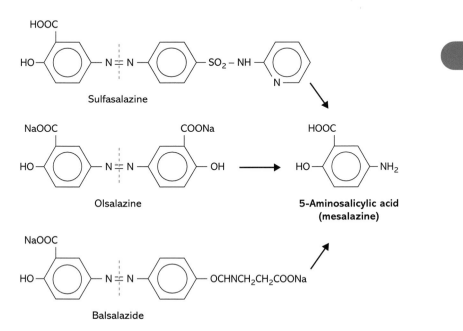

Figure 4.1 Chemistry of 5-aminosalicylate (5-ASA) preparations.

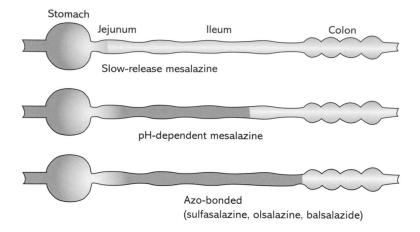

Figure 4.2 Intestinal release profiles of 5-aminosalicylate (5-ASA) formulations (see Table 4.2). There is some variability in the site of release of the various formulations depending on, for example, the precise pH at which 5-ASA is released from different pH-dependent preparations, intestinal intraluminal pH and intestinal transit rate.

may be more effective than those from which 5-ASA is released more proximally. Patients using sulfasalazine in the long term should also be prescribed folic acid to prevent folate deficiency: this may also help to reduce the risk of colonic cancer in chronic extensive ulcerative colitis.

Although mesalazine preparations are moderately effective in active Crohn's disease, the evidence for the usefulness of aminosalicylates in the prevention of symptomatic relapse of quiescent Crohn's disease is equivocal (see Chapter 6).

Side effects. Although better tolerated than sulfasalazine, the newer 5-ASA formulations (Table 4.2) may cause rash, headache, nausea, diarrhea, exacerbation of ulcerative colitis, pancreatitis and/or blood dyscrasias in up to 5% of patients (Table 4.3). Interstitial nephritis has been associated very rarely (about 1 in 500 patients) with mesalazine, while watery diarrhea due to active small-intestinal secretion occurs in about 5% of patients given olsalazine. This can usually be avoided by taking the drug with meals.

Monitoring treatment. Patients taking sulfasalazine require regular (every 3–6 months) blood counts, and serum folate and liver-function tests. Patients receiving any 5-ASA preparation should have occasional (e.g. annual) checks of their serum urea and creatinine concentrations.

Contraindications. All 5-ASAs should be avoided in patients with a history of hypersensitivity to salicylates, including aspirin, or with serious renal impairment. In addition, sulfasalazine should not be given to patients with sulfonamide sensitivity, porphyria or glucose-6-phosphate dehydrogenase deficiency.

Antibiotics
Metronidazole

Pharmacology and mechanism of action. Metronidazole is a nitroimidazole compound with antimicrobial actions against gut anaerobes and protozoa. It also has immunomodulatory effects in vitro. The oral preparation is the most widely used in IBD.

Indications and side effects. Metronidazole, 800 mg/day orally, has moderate benefit in ileocolonic, but not small-bowel, Crohn's disease and in preventing recurrence after ileal resection. Despite the lack of data from controlled trials, it is commonly used in perianal Crohn's disease too. It is also sometimes given in combination with ciprofloxacin in refractory Crohn's disease. Metronidazole has no primary therapeutic role in ulcerative colitis. Treatment in Crohn's disease must be given for up to 3 months, but may be confounded by nausea, vomiting, an unpleasant taste in the mouth and/or patients' unwillingness to abstain from alcohol during this time. The most serious side effect is peripheral neuropathy. This is dose-related, occurs much more often during long-term treatment with 20 mg/kg/day than with 10 mg/kg/day and is not always reversible when treatment ends.

Other antibiotics. Limited data suggest that oral tobramycin and trimethoprim–sulfamethoxazole could improve outcome in acute severe ulcerative colitis. However, most gastroenterologists restrict the use of broad-spectrum antibiotics to prophylaxis against bacteremia and endotoxic shock in severely ill patients with acute severe colitis.

Results from preliminary trials have suggested therapeutic roles for clarithromycin (sometimes in combination with rifabutin) and ciprofloxacin in Crohn's disease, the latter particularly for perianal disease. Like metronidazole, clarithromycin has some immunomodulatory effects in vitro. Antibiotics such as amoxicillin, trimethoprim, ciprofloxacin and metronidazole are sometimes useful for the treatment of diarrhea or steatorrhea due to bacterial overgrowth in patients with small-bowel Crohn's disease.

Immunomodulatory drugs

Immunomodulatory agents currently used in the treatment of IBD include azathioprine and its active metabolite, 6-mercaptopurine (6-MP), and, less often, ciclosporin and methotrexate.

Azathioprine and 6-MP. Azathioprine is a prodrug that undergoes rapid conversion to 6-MP; both are imidazole purine analogs. The doses most commonly used in IBD are 2.0 and 1.0 mg/kg/day, respectively (Table 4.4). Both drugs are currently used only in oral formulations, and take up to 4 months to exert their clinical benefit. Intravenous azathioprine does not, unfortunately, accelerate the response in active IBD.

Homozygous deficiency of 6-thiopurine methyltransferase (6-TPMT), an enzyme responsible for the safe metabolism of azathioprine and 6-MP, occurs in about 0.2% of the population. This deficiency is likely to account for some of the serious untoward effects that can occur with these drugs. An assay to predict the response of individual patients to treatment with these drugs exists, but is not yet widely available, although its use is growing.

Mechanism of action. The precise mechanism of action of azathioprine and 6-MP is not known, but they appear to modify the immune response by inhibiting DNA synthesis in T lymphocytes. Azathioprine has anti-inflammatory and antibacterial as well as immunomodulatory effects.

Indications. Azathioprine and 6-MP are used predominantly as steroid-sparing agents in patients with steroid-dependent or steroid-refractory IBD. They may also have special roles in accelerating

TABLE 4.4

Azathioprine and 6-MP in inflammatory bowel disease

Preparations

Oral	Azathioprine (2.0–2.5 mg/kg/day), 6-MP (1.0–1.5 mg/kg/day)

Indications	Steroid-dependent or -refractory ulcerative colitis and Crohn's disease Fistulating and perianal Crohn's disease

Side effects

General	Nausea, vomiting, headache, arthralgia, fever, rash, abdominal pain
Blood	Agranulocytosis, thrombocytopenia, macrocytosis
Infections	Opportunistic including cytomegalovirus, herpes zoster
Hepatobiliary	Cholestatic hepatitis, acute pancreatitis
Malignancy	Lymphoma, skin (possibly)

Monitoring	Every 2 weeks for the first 2 months, then every 2–3 months: blood count, liver-function tests
Contraindications	Pregnancy (relative contraindication) 6-Thiopurine methyltransferase (6-TPMT) deficiency Concurrent allopurinol
Mechanism of action	Inhibition of T-cell DNA synthesis

6-MP, 6-mercaptopurine.

remission and healing ileal lesions when given in combination with prednisolone in active Crohn's disease, and in fistulating Crohn's disease, particularly perianal disease.

Side effects. Up to 20% of patients cannot tolerate azathioprine because of its side effects (Table 4.4). In about half of these patients, a switch to 6-MP may avert these problems. More seriously, both drugs cause acute pancreatitis in about 3% of patients. Other potentially serious side effects of dose-dependent bone-marrow depression (particularly in the first few weeks of treatment: 2% of patients) and cholestatic hepatitis necessitate regular blood monitoring (see below). There is an increased risk of infections, particularly a serious form of glandular fever. Very long-term use, as in transplant patients, may yet prove to increase the risk of malignancy. Indeed, white patients taking azathioprine or 6-MP should avoid excessive exposure to sunlight because of the risk of skin cancer.

Monitoring treatment. Patients started on azathioprine or 6-MP should have blood counts every 2 weeks for the first 2 months of therapy to check for incipient bone-marrow depression. Thereafter, white-cell count, platelet count and liver-function tests should be performed every 2–3 months.

Contraindications. Although the outcome of accidental pregnancies has been satisfactory (see Chapter 8), azathioprine and 6-MP should, if possible, be avoided in patients likely to conceive. Patients receiving allopurinol should not be given either drug because the former inhibits xanthine oxidase, thus reducing metabolism of azathioprine and 6-MP.

Ciclosporin. This is a fungus-derived cyclic undecapeptide. Intravenous therapy is usually given initially in active disease, replaced after a few days with the oral preparation (Neoral). Recent reports suggest that a lower dose of 2 mg/kg/day (i.v.) is as effective as, and probably safer than, the initially recommended dose of 4 mg/kg/day (i.v.). Close monitoring of whole blood concentrations is used to adjust ciclosporin dosage. The target levels depend on the method used for analysis and on the route of administration (Table 4.5). Because ciclosporin is metabolized via the cytochrome P450 enzyme system, grapefruit juice and drugs that inhibit this enzyme system should be used with caution. However, drugs that *induce* the cytochrome P450 system decrease blood levels of ciclosporin (Table 4.5).

Mechanism of action. Ciclosporin reduces helper and cytotoxic T-cell function and proliferation by inhibiting interleukin-2 (IL-2) gene transcription.

TABLE 4.5

Ciclosporin in inflammatory bowel disease

Preparations

Oral	Neoral, 5 mg/kg/day
Intravenous	2–4 mg/kg/day by continuous infusion

Indications Steroid-refractory acute severe ulcerative colitis (intravenous then oral)

Side effects

General	Nausea, vomiting, headache
Renal	Interstitial nephritis
Infection	Opportunistic, including *Pneumocystis carinii* pneumonia
Neurological	Epileptic fits, paresthesiae, myopathy
Cardiovascular	Hypertension
Skin	Hypertrichosis, gingival hypertrophy
Metabolic	Hyperkalemia, hypomagnesemia, hyperuricemia
Liver	Cholestatic hepatitis
Malignancy	Lymphoma

Monitoring

Pretreatment	Serum urea and creatinine, potassium, magnesium, cholesterol, urate, liver function
On treatment	Blood ciclosporin concentrations: aim for 250–400 ng/mL for intravenous, and trough 150–300 ng/mL for oral ciclosporin Serum urea and creatinine, potassium, magnesium, urate, liver function Blood pressure

Contraindications

Pregnancy, lactation	Renal impairment, hypertension, infection, epilepsy, malignancy
Disease	Low serum cholesterol or magnesium, high potassium

(CONTINUED)

TABLE 4.5 (CONTINUED)

Contraindications (continued)

Biochemical	Coadministration of cytochrome P450 inhibitors (grapefruit juice, erythromycin, oral contraceptives, fluconazole, calcium-channel and proton-pump inhibitors)
Drugs	Coadministration of cytochrome P450 inducers (phenytoin, barbiturates, rifampicin, carbamazepine)
Mechanism of action	Inhibition of IL-2 gene transcription leading to inhibition of helper and cytotoxic T-cell function and proliferation

IL-2, interleukin-2.

Indications. Initial enthusiasm for intravenous ciclosporin in active Crohn's disease and ciclosporin enemas in distal ulcerative colitis was not justified by later reports. The only current indication for ciclosporin in IBD is as an adjunctive treatment in steroid-refractory acute severe ulcerative colitis (see Chapter 5).

Side effects and monitoring. The most serious side effects of ciclosporin are:

- opportunistic infections (occurring in 20% of patients), such as *Pneumocystis carinii* pneumonia, for which coadministration of prophylactic trimethoprim–sulfamethoxazole may be advisable
- renal impairment, including a 20% reduction in glomerular filtration rate in most patients and, in 25% of patients, an interstitial nephritis that is not always reversible when treatment stops
- hypertension (30% of patients)
- hepatotoxicity (up to 20% of patients)
- epileptic fits (3% of patients) due to penetration of the blood–brain barrier by Cremophor, a lipid-soluble vehicle for intravenous ciclosporin; the fits are confined to patients with low serum cholesterol and/or magnesium concentrations, and do not occur with oral ciclosporin.

Long-term oral use of ciclosporin, for which there is no clear indication yet in IBD, may predispose to lymphoma. The side effects of the drug will prevent it ever becoming widely used for IBD. Its use demands frequent monitoring of ciclosporin blood levels and serum biochemistry.

Methotrexate

Mechanism of action. Methotrexate acts predominantly by inhibiting the enzymes that metabolize folic acid. At high doses, the main enzyme affected is dihydrofolate reductase, with consequent inhibition of RNA, DNA and protein synthesis. At the lower doses used to treat Crohn's disease, the anti-inflammatory and immunomodulatory effects of methotrexate are likely to result from inhibition of other folate-dependent enzymes.

Indications. Given weekly as a 25 mg intramuscular injection, methotrexate improves symptoms and reduces steroid requirements in chronically active, steroid-dependent Crohn's disease. An intramuscular dose of 15 mg/week maintains remission in such patients, but the efficacy of lower and/or oral doses is not yet clear. Most gastroenterologists resort first to a thiopurine rather than to methotrexate in steroid-resistant or steroid-dependent patients with Crohn's disease. Methotrexate has not been found to be beneficial in ulcerative colitis.

Side effects necessitate discontinuation of methotrexate in up to 20% of patients. Nausea, vomiting, stomatitis and diarrhea are the most common. As with other immunosuppressive agents, there is an increase in opportunistic infections and bone-marrow depression. These side effects are reduced by coadministration of folic acid, which does not compromise the therapeutic efficacy of methotrexate. Hepatic fibrosis and pneumonitis are the most serious side effects of long-term therapy with methotrexate in patients with psoriasis and rheumatoid arthritis, but they appear to be less common in those with Crohn's disease.

Monitoring treatment. The risk of bone-marrow depression necessitates weekly blood counts for the first 4 weeks, and thereafter every 1–2 months. Folic acid should also be coadministered at a dose of 1–5 mg/day. Liver-function tests, including albumin, should be monitored every 1–2 months. Liver biopsy is probably unnecessary, except in patients with persistently abnormal liver-function tests or after a cumulative dose of more than 5 g. Unexplained shortness of breath or coughing necessitates a chest X-ray and blood gas and lung function tests, particularly measurement of carbon monoxide diffusing capacity.

Contraindications. Pregnancy and conception should be avoided within 6 months of the treatment of either partner, because methotrexate is teratogenic. Breastfeeding is also contraindicated. Coadministration of other antifolate agents, such as trimethoprim–sulfamethoxazole, may increase the toxic effects of methotrexate on the bone marrow, as may NSAIDs, penicillin, old age and renal impairment. To reduce the risk of hepatotoxicity, methotrexate should not be prescribed to patients who drink more than seven units of alcohol per week, weigh over 40% more than their recommended weight for height, or have diabetes mellitus.

Modulation of cytokine activity

Recognition of altered cytokine expression in IBD (see Chapter 1) has prompted trials using anti-tumor necrosis factor α (anti-TNFα) antibody, interleukin-10 (IL-10), IL-11, IL-1 receptor antagonist, IL-12 antibody, interferon-α and interferon-β. Of these, only the first has reached clinical use. In the long term, it is likely that a range of other cytokine-based therapies will enter clinical practice, at least in patients with refractory IBD. These may include gene transfer techniques to induce intestinal mucosal production of anti-inflammatory cytokines, such as IL-4 and IL-10.

Anti-TNFα antibodies. The anti-TNFα antibody preparation infliximab, a mouse–human chimeric antibody, was launched in the USA in 1998 and in the UK and Europe in 1999. Although the merits of infliximab require further clarification with respect to its efficacy, safety and cost, there is little doubt that this new biological therapy represents an important advance for patients with refractory or fistulous Crohn's disease. Reassurance is needed that repeated use of the drug will not lead to serious adverse effects as a result of host–antibody induction or of immunosuppression with consequent infection or malignancy (see below). In the future, it is likely that anti-TNFα antibodies will be replaced by non-protein, small-molecule drugs that prevent the production or actions of TNF.

Pharmacology. Infliximab is administered as single or, to obtain a more prolonged response, multiple intravenous infusions at intervals of 8–15 weeks, each infusion being given over 2 hours. The recommended dose is 5 mg/kg per infusion, and the cost is about \$1800/£1200/€2000 per infusion.

Mechanism of action. The antibody appears to act by binding not only to free TNFα but also to surface-bound TNFα on activated T cells, leading to their apoptosis. The net result is downregulation of the cytokine cascade (see Chapter 1).

Indications. Intravenous infusions of infliximab often induce remission in active, otherwise refractory Crohn's disease, and heal perianal and other fistulas in Crohn's disease (see Chapter 6). Several studies indicate its efficacy in active ulcerative colitis, but its use in this disease is not yet licensed. Anti-TNFα antibody may prove useful in minimizing steroid usage and in preventing growth retardation in children with active Crohn's disease, but uncertainties about its safety necessitate careful control of its use in this age group.

The effects of infliximab in adults with severe, complicated Crohn's disease are impressive, mucosal lesions sometimes healing completely. Coprescription of azathioprine, 6-MP or methotrexate appears to prolong the response to infliximab, possibly by reducing the development of antibodies to infliximab (ATI) and subsequent hypersensitivity reactions (see below). In the future, the selection of patients for treatment with anti-TNFα antibody may depend not only on their disease phenotype (e.g. fistulating disease), but also on their genotype. For example, preliminary evidence suggests that patients with Crohn's disease who are positive for pANCA and have particular TNFα microsatellite haplotypes show a poor response to infliximab.

Side effects. Common side effects associated with the infusion itself include headache, rash, nausea and fever (Table 4.6). These are usually mild and respond to antihistamines. However, anaphylaxis may occur, so antihistamines, adrenaline and corticosteroids should be on hand when infusions are given. Repeat infusions of infliximab after an

TABLE 4.6

Anti-TNFα antibody (infliximab) in inflammatory bowel disease

Preparations

Intravenous	Remicade, 5 mg/kg per infusion

Indications   Steroid-dependent or -refractory active Crohn's disease
Fistulating Crohn's disease
Steroid-dependent/-refractory ulcerative colitis
(unlicensed)
Pyoderma gangrenosum (see page 31)
Ankylosing spondylitis (see page 30)

Side effects

General	Headache (20%), nausea (10%), upper respiratory tract infection (10%)
Serious infections	Tuberculosis, *salmonella*, cellulitis, pneumonia
Infusion reactions	Headache, rash, nausea, fever
Intestinal	Obstruction
Autoantibodies	ATI (delayed hypersensitivity) Antibodies to DNA and cardiolipin (lupus syndrome)
Malignancy	Lymphoma
Neurological	Aseptic meningitis, demyelination
Cardiac	Congestive cardiac failure

Monitoring   Recent PPD skin test (Mantoux) and chest X-ray
Pulse, blood pressure, respiration, temperature
during and 1 hour after infusions

Contraindications   Pregnancy (current or planned in next 6 months),
lactation
Active infection
Current or previous malignancy
Strictures or obstructive symptoms
Previous tuberculosis, multiple sclerosis, heart failure
Hypersensitivity to murine proteins

**Mechanism
of action**   Binding of surface-bound T-cell TNF and free TNF

ATI, antibodies to infliximab; PPD, purified protein derivatives; TNF, tumor necrosis factor.

interval of more than 20 weeks increase the risk of developing ATI (formerly known as human antichimeric antibodies or HACA). These may reduce the efficacy of infliximab, and can cause a delayed serum-sickness-like reaction, characterized by myalgia, arthralgia, rash and fever. This reaction responds to prednisolone and analgesics, but may contraindicate further treatment. Intravenous hydrocortisone given prior to infliximab and long-term use of thiopurines or methotrexate may reduce the formation of ATI.

Several infections have been described in patients receiving infliximab, the most serious being tuberculosis. This is disseminated in over 50% of cases and extrapulmonary in about 25%. To date, it has caused more than 100 deaths worldwide. Infliximab can also exacerbate congestive cardiac failure. Possible neurological complications include aseptic meningitis and irreversible demyelination. In patients with pre-existing intestinal strictures, rapid healing by fibrosis may precipitate bowel obstruction.

There are isolated reports of lymphoma in patients receiving infliximab for Crohn's disease or rheumatoid arthritis, but it is not yet clear whether this complication is due to the drug itself, concurrent therapy with immunosuppressive agents or the underlying disease. Although contraindicated in pregnancy (see below), the outcome of unintended pregnancies in patients receiving infliximab for rheumatoid arthritis and Crohn's disease has been reassuring. Antibodies to double-stranded DNA and to cardiolipin have been observed in up to 15% of patients who receive infliximab for Crohn's disease, and a transient lupus syndrome has been reported in those with rheumatoid arthritis.

Contraindications to the use of anti-TNFα antibodies are shown in Table 4.6. Most of these relate to the potential side effects of treatment described above.

Monitoring. To minimize the risk of reactivated, disseminated tuberculosis, patients should have a PPD (Mantoux) skin test and chest X-ray before infusion of anti-TNFα antibodies. Pulse, blood pressure, respiratory rate and temperature measurements should also be taken half-hourly during, and for 1 hour after, treatment to minimize the risk of infusion reactions. Infusions should be carried out in hospitals, where full resuscitation facilities are available, but they may be performed on an outpatient basis.

New therapeutic approaches

Progressive elucidation of the pathogenesis of IBD (Chapter 1) has led to the evaluation (in experimental animal models of IBD and to a lesser extent in humans) of a number of further therapeutic approaches aimed at specific pathophysiological targets (Figure 4.3, Table 4.7). Over the next few years, several of these options are likely to reach the bedside, particularly for patients with disease refractory to current treatments.

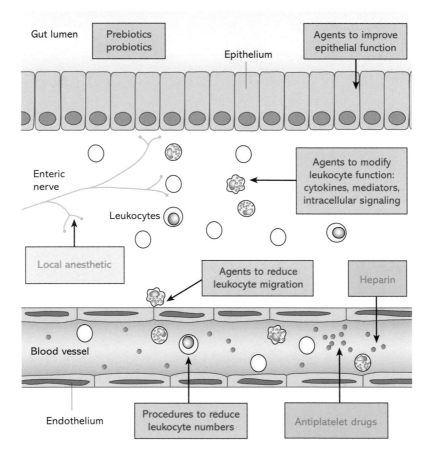

Figure 4.3 Schematic representation of new therapeutic approaches aimed at specific pathophysiological targets.

TABLE 4.7

Potential new treatments for inflammatory bowel disease aimed at specific pathophysiological targets

Target	Agent
Colonic flora	Probiotics (bifidobacteria, *Lactobacillus* spp., non-pathogenic *E. coli*)
	Prebiotics
	Porcine whipworm (*Trichuris suis*) eggs
Epithelium	Short-chain fatty acid enemas,* epidermal growth factor enemas
	Trefoil peptides
	Growth hormone
Leukocytes	
Reduce or increase numbers	Apheresis, anti-CD4 antibodies, bone-marrow or stem-cell transplant, granulocyte colony-stimulating factor
Reduce migration	Adhesion molecule antibodies (nataluzimab) or antisense oligonucleotides (ICAM-1)
Modify intracellular signaling	PPAR-γ agonist, MAP kinase inhibitor
Cytokines	
Reduce proinflammatory cytokines	NF-κB antisense oligonucleotide
Antagonize inflammatory cytokines	Infliximab,* anti-IL-12 antibodies, IL-1 receptor antagonist
Increase anti-inflammatory cytokines	IL-10, interferon-α or -β, IL-11, TGF-β, IL-4 gene therapy
Mediators	Cytoprotective prostaglandins
	Cox-2 inhibition
	Synthesis inhibitors and receptor antagonists of leukotrienes, thromboxanes
	Antioxidants
	Inducible NOS inhibition

(CONTINUED)

TABLE 4.7 (CONTINUED)

Mediators (continued)

	Fish oil (eicosapentaenoic acid, EPA)
	Metalloproteinase inhibitors
Vasculature	Heparin
Enteric nerves	Local anesthetics (lignocaine, ropivercaine enemas)*
Unknown targets	Nicotine (ulcerative colitis),* stopping smoking (Crohn's disease)*

*Current or imminent option (see Table 4.6).

Cox, cyclo-oxygenase; ICAM-1, intercellular adhesion molecule; IL, interleukin; MAP, mitogen-activated protein; NF-κB, nuclear transcription factor κB; NOS, nitric oxide synthase; PPAR, peroxisome-proliferator-activated receptor; TGF, transforming growth factor.

Complementary and alternative therapy

The terms 'complementary' and 'alternative' medicine denote theories and practices in medicine that deviate from conventional ones. The former applies to adjunctive therapies, while the latter applies to treatments that are used instead of standard management. The combined term comprises a heterogeneous range of diagnostic and therapeutic procedures, ranging from traditional practices such as acupuncture, traditional Chinese medicine, homeopathy and herbal medicine, to more modern complementary practices such as aromatherapy and reflexology. Indeed, we suggest that the term 'comprehensive' therapy might be more appropriate than 'alternative' or 'complementary' therapy.

Current usage. Recent surveys have shown that up to 50% of people in the Western world use complementary therapies. Indeed, approximately half of patients with gastrointestinal disorders, including IBD, have used complementary therapies, most commonly herbal remedies. The widespread use of such therapies in IBD is likely to be related to the chronic and refractory nature of the disease, and has been linked with poor quality of life in terms of psychosocial functioning.

Efficacy. Limited data suggest that aloe vera, *Boswellia serrata* and some traditional Chinese medicines may be effective in ulcerative colitis, but there are no data on the efficacy of complementary therapies in Crohn's disease. Despite the difficulties in evaluating complementary medicine, in view of the widespread use of complementary approaches by patients with IBD, it is essential that efforts are made to assess scientifically the efficacy and safety of, at least, the most frequently used therapies.

Side effects. While it is unlikely that therapies such as reflexology will have direct adverse effects, the same cannot be said of herbal therapies: adverse effects have included fatal liver toxicity as well as irreversible renal failure. The interaction of herbal therapies with conventional drugs needs further clarification. In the context of IBD, however, St John's wort reduces blood levels of ciclosporin by enhancing the activity of cytochrome P450 enzymes, while gingko, ginger and devil's claw reduce the absorption of orally administered iron.

Perhaps more importantly, complementary and alternative therapies may be associated with indirect adverse effects. For example, patients who initially consult an alternative practitioner may suffer from misdiagnosis, while others may delay or forego appropriate conventional options in favor of ineffective unconventional ones.

There is an urgent need for further scientific assessment of the benefits and dangers of complementary therapies. Herbal preparations, in particular, should require licensing by an independent national body in order to improve their quality and safety, while claims of efficacy should be validated by controlled trials. The general public, pharmacists and doctors need to be aware of the direct and indirect risks associated with the use of complementary therapies.

Key points – drug treatment

- Treatment for IBD has improved substantially, owing to new formulations and better use of conventional drugs, including corticosteroids, aminosalicylates, antibiotics and immunomodulatory agents.
- Anti-TNFα antibodies (infliximab) represent an important advance for patients with refractory or fistulous Crohn's disease, although reassurance is needed that repeated use of the drug will not lead to serious adverse effects.
- Treatment of IBD is likely to improve further with the advent of new biological therapies arising from improved understanding of the pathogenesis of the disease.
- Complementary and alternative therapies are widely used by patients with IBD, but there are insufficient data on their efficacy and safety.

Key references

Faubion WA Jr., Loftus EV Jr., Harmsen WS et al. The natural history of corticosteroid therapy for inflammatory bowel disease: a population-based study. *Gastroenterology* 2001;121:255–60.

Feagan BG, Rochon J, Fedorak RN et al. Methotrexate for the treatment of Crohn's disease. The North American Crohn's Study Group Investigators. *N Engl J Med* 1995; 332:292–7.

Greenberg GR, Feagan BG, Martin F et al. Oral budesonide for active Crohn's disease. *N Engl J Med* 1994; 331:836–41.

Hanauer SB. Drug therapy: inflammatory bowel disease. *N Engl J Med* 1996;334:841–8.

Hanauer SB, Feagan BG, Lichtenstein GR et al. Maintenance infliximab for Crohn's disease: the ACCENT 1 randomised trial. *Lancet* 2002;359: 1541–9.

Langmead L, Rampton DS. Herbal treatment in gastrointestinal and liver disease – benefits and dangers. *Aliment Pharmacol Ther* 2001; 15:1239–52.

Lichtiger S, Present DH, Kornbluth A et al. Cyclosporine in severe ulcerative colitis refractory to steroid therapy. *N Engl J Med* 1994;330: 1841–5.

Pearson DC, May GR, Fick GH et al. Azathioprine and 6-mercaptopurine in Crohn's disease: a meta-analysis. *Ann Intern Med* 1995;122:132–42.

Present DH, Rutgeerts P, Targan S et al. Infliximab for the treatment of fistulas in patients with Crohn's disease. *N Engl J Med* 1999;340: 1398–405.

Sandborn WJ, Targan SR. Biologic therapy of inflammatory bowel disease. *Gastroenterology* 2002;122:1592–608.

Shanahan F. Inflammatory bowel disease: immunodiagnostics, immunotherapeutics, and ecotherapeutics. *Gastroenterology* 2001;120:622–35.

The management of patients with ulcerative colitis, as for Crohn's disease, comprises general measures, supportive treatment and specific pharmacological and surgical therapies. The aims of treatment are to induce and then maintain remission.

General measures
The general principles of management of IBD are summarized in Table 5.1.

Explanation and psychosocial support. Patients with newly diagnosed ulcerative colitis need a full explanation from their doctor (and, if available, their specialist IBD nurse) about their disease and its implications. This process can be facilitated by the written information and other services provided by patient support groups (for a list of addresses, see the section at the back of this book entitled 'Useful resources'). The services offered by such groups include:
- educational literature, websites and helplines
- lecture and discussion meetings at which patients and their families can share their problems
- specialist counseling for individuals with particular difficulties relating to their illness.

These groups can also direct patients to appropriate social agencies to help with employment problems, and to insurance companies for life, travel and motor insurance. Lastly, large patient support groups can act as a political pressure group to help maximize accessibility of healthcare services to patients with both kinds of IBD, and play a major role in generating funds for research.

Hospital care. Patients with ulcerative colitis are best managed, whether as outpatients or during admission to hospital, by specialist gastroenterological medical, surgical, nursing and dietetic staff working in close collaboration, with access to stoma therapists and, if possible,

TABLE 5.1

Principles of the management of inflammatory bowel disease

General measures

Explanation, psychosocial support
- physicians, specialist nurses
- patient support groups

Specialist multidisciplinary hospital care
- monitoring disease activity, nutrition, therapy
- checking for extraintestinal complications
- colonoscopic cancer surveillance

Supportive treatment

Dietary and nutritional advice

Drugs
- antidiarrheal agents (not in active colitis)
- colestyramine (ileal disease or resection for Crohn's disease)
- hematinics (iron, folate)
- vitamins, electrolytes
- osteoporosis prophylaxis and treatment
- heparin, administered subcutaneously (inpatients with active IBD)

Drugs to avoid
- antidiarrheal drugs (in active colitis)
- non-essential NSAIDs, antibiotics, delayed-release drugs

Specific treatment (according to presentation)

Drugs
- corticosteroids
- aminosalicylates
- immunomodulatory drugs (azathioprine/6-MP, ciclosporin, methotrexate – Crohn's disease only)
- antibiotics
- cytokine therapy (infliximab – Crohn's disease only)
- other

Nutritional therapy (Crohn's disease only)

- liquid formula diet

Surgery

6-MP, 6-mercaptopurine; NSAID, non-steroidal anti-inflammatory drug.

a trained counselor. Specialist outpatient IBD clinics are the best way of providing patients with the necessary clinical expertise in the form of joint medical–surgical consultations with open access for prompt review in the event of relapse. Such clinics also offer:

- continuity of care
- appropriate clinical, endoscopic and laboratory monitoring of the disease and its treatment
- training for doctors and nurses
- a sufficient patient base for clinical trials.

Most primary care physicians have fewer than 5 patients with IBD under their care; this limited experience of the disease means that they should not generally be expected to take primary responsibility for the long-term management of either ulcerative colitis or Crohn's disease. However, some patients with stable, inactive and limited disease can be followed safely by their family doctor. This arrangement is dependent on appropriate shared-care guidelines as well as prompt open access to the hospital IBD clinic when necessary.

Dietary advice and nutritional support. Patients with ulcerative colitis do not usually need specific dietary advice, although a few (less than 5%) may find their condition improves if they avoid cows' milk, and some with proctitis and proximal constipation may benefit from fiber supplementation.

Specific nutritional deficiencies are less common in ulcerative colitis than in Crohn's disease, but should be corrected as necessary with appropriate supplements. Sick inpatients who are malnourished often need enteral and occasionally total parenteral nutrition. However, there is no evidence that enteral nutrition is itself an effective primary therapy in active ulcerative colitis, in contrast to small-bowel Crohn's disease.

Drugs. Iron (see below) and folic acid supplements are sometimes needed, as are appropriate drugs for incipient or established osteoporosis (see Chapter 2). Subcutaneous heparin is recommended for patients admitted with active ulcerative colitis to reduce the risk of arterial and venous thrombosis.

Drugs to avoid. Antidiarrheal (loperamide, codeine phosphate, diphenoxylate), opioid analgesic, antispasmodic and anticholinergic drugs should be avoided in active ulcerative colitis as they may provoke acute colonic dilation. NSAIDs, and occasionally antibiotics, may provoke relapse of ulcerative colitis (see Chapter 1), and should not be used unless essential.

Treatment of active ulcerative colitis

Treatment is determined by:
- the extent of disease
- the severity of the attack.

Knowledge of the extent of disease is particularly important in relation to the feasibility of effective topical therapy, while the severity of the attack defines not only the optimal type and route of therapy, but also whether the patient can be safely treated as an outpatient or needs urgent hospital admission.

Who needs hospital admission? Immediate admission is required for patients with acute severe attacks of ulcerative colitis, defined primarily by clinical features (see Chapter 2). These include six or more bloody diarrheal stools daily, pyrexia and tachycardia (> 90 beats/minute). Such patients will usually be systemically unwell, may be anemic and may have lost weight; in very ill patients there may be abdominal tenderness and/or distension. The decision to admit does not usually depend on the results of blood or other tests of disease severity, though these will often be abnormal (see 'Blood tests', below).

It is also advisable to admit less sick patients who have failed to respond as outpatients to 2 weeks' treatment with oral prednisolone (see 'Active left-sided or extensive ulcerative colitis', below). Since the initial attack of ulcerative colitis is more dangerous than subsequent ones, the threshold for admission should be lowered in patients presenting for the first time with bloody diarrhea.

Inpatient management of acute severe ulcerative colitis

General measures. These patients should be admitted immediately to a gastroenterology ward for close joint medical, surgical and nursing care

(Table 5.2). Early involvement of the nutrition team and of a stoma therapist in patients likely to need surgery is important. All patients undergoing an acute attack of ulcerative colitis need to be kept fully informed of their treatment and its likely outcome; they need to be aware from the outset that they have a one in four chance of needing an urgent colectomy during their admission.

Establishing the diagnosis, extent of disease and its severity requires a carefully targeted history and appropriate investigations (see Chapter 3) in patients presenting for the first time. In patients with established ulcerative colitis, these procedures are required to exclude infection and to assess disease extent (if not already known) and severity.

Clinical evaluation. In patients with established ulcerative colitis, direct questions about stool frequency, consistency and urgency, overt blood content, abdominal pain, malaise, fever and weight loss indicate the severity of the attack (see above, 'Who needs hospital admission?'). External examination should include assessment of general health, pulse rate and temperature, as well as a check for anemia, fluid depletion, weight loss, abdominal tenderness or distension.

The differential diagnosis may also need evaluation in patients presenting with bloody diarrhea for the first time (see Table 3.1). Abrupt onset with fever, vomiting, epidemic or contact history and/or recent foreign travel suggests infective colitis, even in patients with pre-existing ulcerative colitis. Cytomegalovirus (CMV) should be considered, particularly in patients who are known to be immunosuppressed. Antibiotic exposure predisposes to C. *difficile* infection, while NSAIDs may cause either a relapse of established IBD or de novo colitis (which usually remits rapidly on NSAID withdrawal). In patients presenting for the first time, non-smoking or recent cessation of smoking increases the likelihood of ulcerative colitis, while previous abdominal or pelvic irradiation make radiation colitis a strong possibility. Ischemic colitis usually shows sudden onset in older people with other features of vascular disease, and often causes marked abdominal pain as well as bloody diarrhea. The very rare Behçet's enterocolitis may be suggested by a history of cyclical oral and genital ulceration, uveitis, erythema nodosum, pathergy (the

TABLE 5.2

Principles of inpatient management of acute severe ulcerative colitis

General measures

Explanation, psychosocial support
- physicians, specialist nurses
- patient support groups

Specialist multidisciplinary care
- physicians, surgeons, nutrition team, nurses, stoma therapist, counselor

Establishing the diagnosis, extent and severity

Clinical evaluation
Complete blood cell count, ESR, C-reactive protein, albumin, liver-function tests, amebic serology
Stool microscopy, culture, *Clostridium difficile* toxin
Sigmoidoscopy and biopsy
Plain abdominal X-ray
Consider colonoscopy, air or instant contrast enema, leukocyte scan

Monitoring progress

Daily clinical assessment
- abdominal examination (twice daily)
- stool chart
- 4-hourly temperature, pulse

Daily complete blood cell count, ESR, C-reactive protein, urea and electrolytes, albumin
Daily plain abdominal X-ray

Supportive treatment

Intravenous fluids, electrolytes, blood transfusion
Nutritional supplementation
Subcutaneous heparin
Avoid antidiarrheals (codeine, loperamide, diphenoxylate), opiates, NSAIDs
Rolling maneuver (if colon dilating)

(CONTINUED)

TABLE 5.2 (CONTINUED)

Specific treatments

Medical
- intravenous (hydrocortisone or methylprednisolone) then oral corticosteroids (prednisolone)
- continue with oral 5-ASA in patients already taking it; otherwise start when improvement begins
- antibiotics for very sick febrile patients, or when infection is suspected
- for patients not responding to steroids at 4–7 days, consider intravenous then oral ciclosporin (with trimethoprim–sulfamethoxazole prophylaxis) or an infliximab infusion

Surgical (for non-responders at 5–7 days, toxic megacolon, perforation, massive hemorrhage)
- panproctocolectomy with ileoanal pouch or permanent ileostomy
- subtotal colectomy with ileorectal anastomosis (rarely)

5-ASA, 5-aminosalicylate; ESR, erythrocyte sedimentation rate; NSAIDs, non-steroidal anti-inflammatory drugs.

formation of pustules at the site of minor trauma, such as venepuncture) and/or arthropathy.

Blood tests. These are better for establishing the activity of ulcerative colitis than for making the diagnosis or identifying its extent (see Chapter 3). The best laboratory measures of disease activity in ulcerative colitis are hemoglobin, platelet count, ESR, C-reactive protein and serum albumin. For recent travellers, serology as well as stool samples should be requested (for amebiasis, strongyloidiasis and schistosomiasis).

Sigmoidoscopy and rectal biopsy. Cautious rigid or flexible sigmoidoscopy and biopsy in the unprepared patient, and without excessive air insufflation, provides immediate confirmation of active colitis (see Chapter 3 and Figure 1.4). Full colonoscopy may cause colonic perforation and dilation, and should be avoided in acute severe ulcerative colitis.

Plain abdominal X-ray. A plain film at presentation is used to assess disease extent and activity, and to look for dilation (see Chapter 3 and

Figure 3.2). In patients with suspected colonic perforation, diagnosis can be confirmed by erect chest X-ray or a lateral decubitus abdominal film.

Radiolabeled leukocyte scans. ^{99}Tc-HMPAO scanning provides information about disease activity and particularly extent where doubt exists in patients with ulcerative colitis (see Chapter 3, 'Radiolabeled leukocyte scans', and Figure 3.5).

Monitoring progress. Progress is monitored by twice-daily clinical assessment, including:

- abdominal examination, particularly by percussion, for gaseous distension, loss of hepatic dullness (which may indicate free gas in the peritoneal cavity), and peritoneal irritation
- stool chart (recording frequency, consistency, presence of overt blood and urgency)
- 4-hourly measurement of temperature and pulse.

Blood count, ESR, C-reactive protein, routine biochemistry and plain abdominal X-ray should be undertaken daily in sick patients (Table 5.2).

Supportive treatment

Intravenous fluids and blood. Most patients require intravenous fluids and electrolytes, particularly potassium, to replace diarrheal losses. The serum potassium concentration should be maintained at or above 4 mmol/liter, since hypokalemia may predispose to colonic dilation. Blood transfusion is usually recommended if the hemoglobin level falls below 10 g/dL.

Nutritional support. Patients can usually eat normally, with liquid protein and calorie supplements if necessary. Very sick patients, many of whom will undergo surgery, may need enteral or parenteral nutrition.

Anticoagulation. Because active ulcerative colitis is associated with a high risk of venous and arterial thromboembolism, patients should be given prophylactic subcutaneous heparin (e.g. low-molecular-weight heparin, 3000–5000 units daily). Heparin does not appear to increase rectal blood loss, even when given intravenously. Indeed, uncontrolled trials suggest that intravenous heparin may have a primary therapeutic role in acute severe ulcerative colitis (see 'Heparin' below and Table 4.7).

Drugs to avoid. Patients should avoid antidiarrheal (codeine phosphate, loperamide, diphenoxylate), opioid analgesic, antispasmodic and anticholinergic drugs, as well as NSAIDs. If mild pain relief is needed, oral paracetamol appears to be well tolerated, while severe pain suggests colonic dilation or perforation needing urgent evaluation and/or intervention.

Rolling maneuver. In very sick patients, particularly those with clinical and/or radiological evidence of incipient colonic dilation, rolling into the prone or knee–elbow position (Figure 5.1) for 15 minutes every 2 hours may aid in the evacuation of gas from the rectum, deflation of the colon and prevention of toxic megacolon.

Drug therapy. Corticosteroids remain the cornerstone of specific medical treatment for acute severe ulcerative colitis. Aminosalicylates and antibiotics have minor roles. Ciclosporin is useful in some steroid-refractory patients, while the role of heparin remains uncertain. However, oral azathioprine and 6-MP are too slow to work in patients with acute steroid-refractory attacks.

Corticosteroids. Hydrocortisone (300–400 mg/day) or methylprednisolone (40–60 mg/day) are given intravenously. There is no advantage in giving higher doses, although continuous infusion may be more effective than once- or twice-daily boluses. Corticosteroid

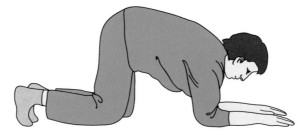

Figure 5.1 Knee–elbow position for rolling maneuver.

drip enemas (e.g. prednisolone, 20 mg, or hydrocortisone, 100 mg in 100–200 mL water given rectally via a soft catheter twice daily with the patient in the left lateral position) are sometimes given in addition to intravenous steroids, but their value is unproven.

About 70% of patients who receive corticosteroids improve substantially in 5–7 days. They are then switched to oral prednisolone (40–60 mg/day), the dose being tapered to zero over 2–3 months. Conventionally, failure to respond to intravenous steroids after 7 days indicates urgent colectomy (see Chapter 7), but the introduction of ciclosporin can now be considered as an alternative (see below).

Aminosalicylates. Aminosalicylates, in full dose, should be continued in patients who are already taking them at the time of admission and are well enough to take oral medication, but these drugs do not have a primary therapeutic effect in acute severe ulcerative colitis. In case patients given aminosalicylates for the first time prove to be allergic to or intolerant of them, initiation of this therapy is best delayed until the patient has improved sufficiently while receiving intravenous steroids to switch to oral treatment (see Tables 4.2 and 4.3).

Antibiotics. The use of antibiotics is usually restricted to very sick febrile patients, or to those in whom an infective component is strongly suspected. Under such circumstances, a combination of antibiotics is often given (e.g. ciprofloxacin or a cephalosporin with metronidazole).

Ciclosporin. Intravenous ciclosporin, 2–4 mg/kg/day for 5 days, followed by oral ciclosporin (Neoral), 5 mg/kg/day, given with continued corticosteroids, averts colectomy in the acute phase in 60%–80% of patients who fail to respond to intravenous steroids given alone for 5–7 days. Oral trimethoprim–sulfamethoxazole may be coprescribed as prophylaxis against *P. carinii* infection. Enthusiasm for this treatment has to be tempered both by the frequency of relapse necessitating colectomy (up to 50%) that follows withdrawal of ciclosporin, and by its serious adverse effects (see Table 4.5) which, in turn, demand frequent monitoring of ciclosporin blood levels and serum biochemistry.

Infliximab. Recent controlled data indicate that after a single infusion of infliximab, 5 mg/kg, colectomy can be avoided in 70% of patients who have failed to improve with intravenous steroids alone.

This response rate closely resembles that with ciclosporin (see above). Further experience with this approach is required before a definitive conclusion can be drawn as to whether ciclosporin or infliximab is the better treatment in patients with steroid-refractory acute severe ulcerative colitis.

Heparin. Anecdotal reports suggest that intravenous heparin can induce remission in acute severe ulcerative colitis. However, limited controlled trials have given conflicting results. Heparin has a variety of anti-inflammatory effects that appear to outweigh its theoretically disadvantageous anticoagulant effects. Indeed, increased rectal bleeding does not appear to be a major problem when intravenous heparin is used in this setting. Nevertheless, the use of heparin requires further evaluation in controlled clinical trials.

Toxic megacolon. As mentioned earlier, the rolling maneuver may help to prevent toxic megacolon in very sick patients (see Figure 5.1). If the intensive treatment outlined in Table 5.2 (including rolling, intravenous antibiotics and a nasogastric tube to aspirate bowel gas and fluids) has not produced improvement in 24–48 hours, and if colonic dilation becomes established, particularly if associated with systemic toxicity, immediate surgery (see Chapter 7) is indicated.

Colonic perforation and massive hemorrhage. After appropriate urgent resuscitation, including intravenous antibiotics and blood transfusion respectively, emergency surgery (see Chapter 7) is required for both of these rare complications. Even with immediate surgical intervention, the mortality of colonic perforation, which can occasionally also occur in patients without colonic dilation, is up to 30%.

Outcome. As indicated above, about 80% of patients with severe ulcerative colitis avoid colectomy in the acute phase when treated with intravenous corticosteroids (and ciclosporin additionally if necessary). Of these, however, over 50% will have had a colectomy for recurrent episodes of active disease before 5 years has elapsed. Mortality of acute severe ulcerative colitis should now be less than 3%.

Active left-sided or extensive ulcerative colitis (mild-to-moderate attack)

The principles of evaluation and management of mild-to-moderate attacks of ulcerative colitis (when the patient is well, with < 6 stools daily) resemble those described above for inpatients (see Table 5.2). These patients, however, can usually be managed as outpatients. Stools should be sent to be checked for infection. In mild attacks of left-sided disease, an oral 5-ASA (see Table 4.2) with twice-daily 5-ASA or steroid enemas may suffice; balsalazide may be more effective and better tolerated than mesalazine in this setting. Often, however, oral prednisolone, 20–60 mg/day (the dose depending on the severity of the attack), is also needed for 2–3 weeks. The dose is then tapered by 5 mg every 5–10 days. Oral iron and/or folate may also be necessary.

Those who do not begin to respond to these measures within 2 weeks (10–40% of patients) or deteriorate often need prompt hospital admission for more intensive management, including intravenous steroids (see above and Table 5.2). An alternative approach in steroid-refractory patients who are not so acutely ill as to require hospital admission, and in whom a response to treatment taking up to 4 months is acceptable, is to introduce oral azathioprine, 2.0–2.5 mg/kg/day, or 6-MP, 1.0–1.5 mg/kg/day, with appropriate laboratory monitoring (see Table 4.4).

Active proctitis

The principles of the management of proctitis resemble those described above for more extensive ulcerative colitis. Management aspects specific to distal disease are outlined below and in Table 5.3.

Establishing the diagnosis. The diagnosis of proctitis, together with its extent and severity, can usually be quickly confirmed by rigid or flexible sigmoidoscopy and biopsy. However, care needs to be taken not to mistake rectal Crohn's disease, cancer, polyps, benign solitary ulcer, hemorrhoids, anal fissure or 'gay bowel' for proctitis. In patients who prove difficult to treat, and depending on the clinical picture, other diagnoses such as irritable bowel syndrome (which

TABLE 5.3

Principles of the treatment of active proctitis

Supportive treatment

Treat proximal constipation with fiber and/or a laxative
(e.g. magnesium hydroxide)

Avoid cows' milk or other specific food (rarely)

Specific treatment

Topical 5-ASA or, as second line, steroids (suppository, liquid or foam
enema)

Oral 5-ASA

Refractory proctitis

Oral or intravenous steroids

Oral azathioprine or 6-MP

Acetarsol suppositories

Other possibilities: ciclosporin, lignocaine or short-chain fatty acid
enemas, nicotine patches or enemas

Surgery: total proctocolectomy

5-ASA, 5-aminosalicylate; 6-MP, 6-mercaptopurine.

may coexist with proctitis), celiac disease, collagenous colitis,
NSAID-induced colitis and 5-ASA intolerance should also be
considered.

Supportive treatment. Rarely, patients benefit from avoiding cows'
milk or other food components that they have noticed provoke
attacks. In patients with proximal constipation, a high-fiber diet,
oral fiber supplements and/or a stool-softening laxative such as
magnesium hydroxide may be helpful. It is conceivable that alleviation
of constipation may improve the symptoms of proctitis, at least in
part, by increasing the delivery of orally administered 5-ASA to the
rectum.

Specific medical treatment. Depending on disease extent, suppositories or enemas of 5-ASA (see Table 4.3) or corticosteroids (see Table 4.1) are inserted once or twice daily until about 2 weeks after bleeding subsides. Suppositories reach about 100 mm from the anal margin, foam enemas 200 mm and liquid enemas, with optimal patient positioning, the splenic flexure. Topical treatment with 5-ASA preparations is more effective than with corticosteroids. Although prednisolone metasulfobenzoate and budesonide enemas suppress adrenal function to a lesser extent than other topical steroids, the choice of product for routine use depends on patient preference in relation to ease of insertion and retention, foam often being favored on both counts.

In patients with recurrent attacks, an oral aminosalicylate (see Table 4.2) is added, in part to initiate subsequent remission maintenance in patients who prefer long-term oral to rectal treatment. Balsalazide and olsalazine, which deliver 5-ASA exclusively to the colon, may be preferable to slow-release or pH-dependent delayed-release aminosalicylates, which release 5-ASA more proximally.

Refractory proctitis

Up to 80% of patients respond in 2–4 weeks to the measures described above for treating active proctitis. In those who do not respond, the diagnosis needs careful confirmation (see above). Alternative approaches in refractory proctitis, which can sometimes be very difficult to treat, include full-dose oral or even intravenous corticosteroids (see above), and oral azathioprine, 2.0–2.5 mg/kg/day, or 6-MP, 1.0–1.5 mg/kg/day. Suppositories containing arsenic (acetarsol) may induce remission in distal disease but, because of the risk of systemic arsenic toxicity, should only be used for short-term management (up to 4 weeks). More experimental options include ciclosporin, short-chain fatty acid or lignocaine enemas, and nicotine patches or enemas (see Table 4.7). None of the enemas listed is commercially available yet, but many hospital pharmacies will prepare them if requested.

Many patients will feel angry about their disease and their doctor's failure to rectify their symptoms; some may need counseling. In exceptional cases, all medical treatments fail, and patients require panproctocolectomy (see Chapter 7). Left-sided colonic resections in ulcerative colitis are too frequently followed by recurrence in the residual colon to be a practical option.

Maintaining remission

5-ASAs. Patients with disease of limited extent and relapses occurring less than once a year may decline maintenance therapy. However, most require an oral aminosalicylate for life (Table 4.2) with appropriate blood checks every 6–12 months (Table 4.3). Such therapy reduces the annual relapse rate to 20–30% from 70–80% with no treatment. Olsalazine may be superior to mesalazine for maintenance therapy, particularly for patients with left-sided disease. To minimize possible systemic side effects, some patients with recurrent attacks of distal disease may prefer topical prophylactic 5-ASA therapy, with enemas or suppositories once or twice daily or even three times weekly.

Azathioprine and 6-MP. In patients who relapse repeatedly despite a 5-ASA in adequate dosage, and/or whenever steroid therapy after acute episodes is withdrawn, oral azathioprine, 2–2.5 mg/kg/day, or 6-MP, 1–1.5 mg/kg/day, carefully monitored (Table 4.4) and given for at least 2 years, is of proven benefit. How long the therapy should be maintained for patients with ulcerative colitis is unclear. It may be prudent to attempt to discontinue it after 4–5 years without relapse.

Infliximab. Two recent similar trials suggest that infusions of infliximab, 5 mg/kg every 8 weeks, maybe useful in maintaining remission in patients with ulcerative colitis that is poorly controlled by steroids and/or thiopurines. Whether the benefit obtained with infliximab in this context outweighs its side effects and justifies its cost (see pages 65–67) is not yet clear.

Surgery. Occasionally, patients continue to have active ulcerative colitis despite all the measures described above. These, particularly if steroid-dependent, require proctocolectomy (Chapter 7).

Follow-up

Patients with well-controlled distal ulcerative colitis can be followed routinely by the primary care physician, subject to referral for colonoscopy at 8–10 years to reassess disease extent in relation to the possible need for cancer surveillance (see below). They should also be referred promptly to a gastroenterologist if they fail to respond to treatment for relapse.

All other patients require periodic review (every 6–12 months if in remission) in a specialized hospital clinic offering immediate open access in the event of relapse. Such arrangements ensure continuity of care and optimal monitoring of the disease, its complications and its treatment. At routine outpatient appointments, disease activity is assessed by questions about bowel habit, quality of life, and time off work; sigmoidoscopy is reserved for patients in whom the history suggests active disease.

Surveillance for colorectal cancer. The increased risk of colorectal cancer in chronic extensive ulcerative colitis (see Chapter 2) has led to the introduction of colonoscopic surveillance programs, in which multiple biopsies from randomly selected sites throughout the colon, and from any raised lesions, are taken every 1–3 years, depending on the duration of the disease, and starting 8–10 years after onset. If these biopsies show the premalignant changes of high-grade epithelial dysplasia (Figure 5.2), colectomy is indicated (Chapter 7).

In patients with confirmed low-grade dysplasia, colectomy or, for those reluctant to have surgery, more frequent colonoscopic surveillance is recommended, because the incidence of cancer in this situation is about 50% in 5 years. Unfortunately, surveillance programs have not been shown to reduce mortality from colonic cancer in ulcerative colitis, in part because about 25% of cancers occur in patients without detected, preceding or associated dysplasia.

Molecular biological techniques (e.g. looking for DNA aneuploidy, p53 heterozygosity) are likely, in due course, to supersede dependence on the colonoscopic detection of dysplasia for the prevention of colorectal cancer in ulcerative colitis.

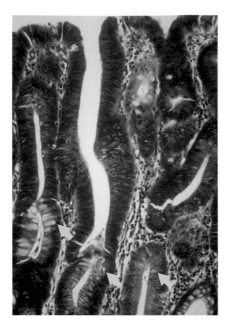

Figure 5.2 Severe epithelial dysplasia in ulcerative colitis, showing glandular distortion, stratification of the epithelium with heaping of nuclei, and nuclear polymorphism and hyperchromaticism. Note the normal crypts at the bottom of the picture (arrowed). Photomicrograph courtesy of Dr RM Feakins, Barts and the London, Queen Mary School of Medicine and Dentistry, London, UK.

Indeterminate colitis

Acute indeterminate colitis, in which the clinical, endoscopic and histological features of the disease do not allow its definite classification as either ulcerative colitis or Crohn's colitis (see Chapter 2), is managed like acute severe ulcerative colitis. However, in patients coming to surgery, it is usually advisable to avoid the immediate formation of an ileoanal pouch, in view of the high risk of pouch failure if the diagnosis proves to be Crohn's disease (see Chapter 7).

Key points – medical management of ulcerative colitis

- The treatment of ulcerative colitis depends on disease extent and severity.
- Active ulcerative colitis is treated primarily with corticosteroids and aminosalicylates, with ciclosporin or surgery for refractory acute severe disease.
- Maintenance of remission in ulcerative colitis is usually achieved with aminosalicylates, although thiopurines are required for patients in whom aminosalicylates are ineffective.
- Patients with ulcerative colitis should participate in decisions about their treatment, particularly in relation to possible surgery.

Key references

Azad-Khan AK, Piris J, Truelove SC. An experiment to determine the active moiety of sulphasalazine. *Lancet* 1977;2:892–5.

Hawthorne AB, Logan RF, Hawkey CJ et al. Randomised controlled trial of azathioprine withdrawal in ulcerative colitis. *BMJ* 1992;305:20–2.

Jarnerot G, Hertervig E, Friis-Liby I et al. Infliximab as rescue therapy in severe to moderately severe ulcerative colitis: a randomised, placebo-controlled study. *Gastroenterology* 2005;128:1805–11.

Kornbluth A, Sachar DB. Ulcerative colitis practice guidelines in adults (update). American College of Gastroenterology, Practice Parameters Committee. *Am J Gastroenterol* 2004;99:1371–85.

Lichtiger S, Present DH, Kornbluth A et al. Cyclosporine in severe ulcerative colitis refractory to steroid therapy. *N Engl J Med* 1994;330:1841–5.

Sutherland L, Roth D, Beck P, Makiyama K. Oral 5-aminosalicylic acid for maintenance of remission in ulcerative colitis. *Cochrane Database Syst Rev* 2002;4:CD000544 (www.thecochranelibrary.com).

Truelove SC, Witts LJ. Cortisone in ulcerative colitis. Final report on a therapeutic trial. *BMJ* 1955;2:1041–8.

Treatment of Crohn's disease not only depends on disease activity and site, as in ulcerative colitis, but also needs to be tailored according to the patient's clinical presentation and its dominant underlying pathological explanation. Inflammation, obstruction, abscess and fistula require different therapeutic approaches, and often need to be distinguished by appropriate investigation before specific treatment is begun. Drug therapy in Crohn's disease is generally less effective than in ulcerative colitis, and dietary and surgical treatment correspondingly more important.

General measures

Explanation, psychosocial support and hospital care. Newly diagnosed patients with Crohn's disease, as with ulcerative colitis, need a full explanation of their illness, preferably assisted by the written information provided by patient support groups (see Chapter 5, Table 5.1 and the 'Useful resources' section). A substantial minority of patients are sufficiently disturbed psychologically by the chronically disabling nature of their illness to need more formal psychosocial help. As with ulcerative colitis, out- and inpatient care is best undertaken by a specialist multidisciplinary hospital team.

Dietary advice and nutritional support. All patients should be carefully assessed in relation to their nutritional intake and status, the latter clinically by measurement of weight, height and then body mass index (BMI = weight [kg]/height [m]^2; normal BMI > 20).

Patients with stricturing small-bowel Crohn's disease should avoid high-residue foods (e.g. citrus fruit, nuts, sweetcorn, uncooked vegetables) that might cause bolus obstruction. Special dietary and nutritional modifications are needed for patients with extensive small-bowel Crohn's disease, or short bowel syndrome (see Chapter 2). Sick inpatients may need enteral or parenteral nutrition to restore nutritional deficits, while liquid formula diets provide a primary therapy option for some patients with active small-bowel Crohn's disease (see below).

Non-specific drugs. Diarrhea in Crohn's disease has a number of different causes, each requiring a different therapeutic approach (see Table 2.1). Codeine phosphate and loperamide are often useful for the symptomatic control of diarrhea that is due to active disease or previous bowel resection. As in active ulcerative colitis, however, they should be avoided in active Crohn's colitis in case they provoke colonic dilation.

Colestyramine (cholestyramine), 4 g one to three times daily, is often helpful in patients with Crohn's disease complicated by bile-salt-induced diarrhea as a result of extensive terminal ileal disease or resection (see Chapter 7, 'Bile-salt malabsorption'). By binding bile salts, colestyramine may, however, exacerbate or induce steatorrhea and malabsorption of fat-soluble vitamins; it may also directly bind with and prevent the absorption of other drugs, and should not, therefore, be given simultaneously with other therapies.

Hematinics (iron, folate, vitamin B_{12}), calcium, magnesium, zinc and fat-soluble vitamins (A, D, E and K) may be needed for the replacement of particular deficiencies, as may appropriate drugs for incipient or established osteoporosis (see Chapter 2). Subcutaneous heparin to reduce the risk of arterial and venous thrombosis is recommended in patients admitted with active Crohn's disease.

Drugs to avoid. NSAIDs may precipitate relapse of Crohn's disease and should, if possible, be avoided. Likewise, in patients with small-bowel stricturing due to Crohn's disease, delayed-release drugs should not be prescribed in case they cause bolus obstruction. Anecdotal evidence suggests that iron salts can exacerbate relapses, and their prescription is best postponed until remission has been achieved. In patients who are frequently hospitalized because of pain, use of opiates should be minimized to avoid narcotic addiction.

Treatment of active Crohn's disease

Who needs hospital admission? The heterogeneous presentation of Crohn's disease makes assessment of disease activity more complicated than in ulcerative colitis. For clinical trials, a large number of multifactorial clinical and/or laboratory-based scoring systems, such as the Crohn's Disease Activity Index (CDAI), has been devised, but none is suitable for ordinary clinical use. The working definitions of the American College of Gastroenterology (Table 6.1) are more practical. Many patients with active Crohn's disease can be looked after as outpatients, but those with moderate to severe and severe to fulminant disease need prompt, and in the latter instance immediate, hospital admission. In patients with Crohn's colitis, indications for admission resemble those for acute severe ulcerative colitis (see Chapter 5).

General measures. As for ulcerative colitis, patients with active Crohn's disease should be looked after by a multidisciplinary team with special expertise in IBD in a specialist gastroenterology clinic or ward (see

TABLE 6.1

American College of Gastroenterology's working definition of disease activity in Crohn's disease

Activity	Features
Remission	Asymptomatic patients
Mild to moderate	Outpatients able to take oral nutrition, with symptoms but no fluid depletion, fever, abdominal tenderness, painful mass or obstruction
Moderate to severe	Patients who have failed to respond to treatment of mild to moderate disease, or those with more prominent symptoms including fever, weight loss >10%, abdominal pain or tenderness (without rebound), intermittent nausea or vomiting (without obstructive findings) or anemia
Severe to fulminant	Patients with persisting symptoms despite outpatient oral steroids, or those with high fever, persistent vomiting, intestinal obstruction, rebound tenderness, cachexia or abscess

Adapted from Hanauer SB, Meyers S. *Am J Gastroenterol* 2001;96:635–43.

Table 5.1). Options for treatment (medical, nutritional, surgical) are wider than in ulcerative colitis, and it is essential that the patient with Crohn's disease is kept fully informed about his or her illness, and takes a place at the center of the therapeutic decision-making process.

Establishing the diagnosis, clinicopathological problem and severity. For many patients, the diagnosis of Crohn's disease and identification of its principal site will have been made before he or she presents with a relapse. Investigations, therefore, are directed primarily at clarifying the dominant clinicopathological process so as to optimize subsequent treatment. In individuals presenting acutely for the first time, the diagnosis must be established (Table 6.2; see also Tables 3.1–3.4).

Clinical evaluation. Symptoms of active terminal ileal and ileocecal Crohn's disease are described in Chapter 2. Where the diagnosis of Crohn's disease has not yet been made, acute appendicitis with a mass may be particularly hard to differentiate from Crohn's disease, except with laparoscopy or laparotomy. In elderly patients presenting de novo, cecal carcinoma and lymphoma need careful consideration, while in some ethnic groups, for example South Asians, ileocecal tuberculosis must be excluded.

In Crohn's colitis, diarrhea is a more prominent symptom than pain; questions to be asked of previously undiagnosed patients are outlined in the section on acute severe ulcerative colitis in Chapter 5. External abdominal or perianal fistulas are usually clinically obvious, but direct questions may be necessary to identify enterovesical or enterovaginal fistulas.

Blood tests. As in ulcerative colitis, the main value of blood tests is in assessing and monitoring disease activity, which is related directly to the platelet count, ESR and C-reactive protein, and inversely to serum albumin. However, in very sick patients, particularly those with extensive small-bowel disease and steatorrhea, there may be laboratory evidence of malnutrition and malabsorption (anemia, low serum iron, folate, B_{12}, albumin, calcium, magnesium, zinc, essential fatty acids). A raised neutrophil count suggests intra-abdominal abscess, but corticosteroids also cause leukocytosis by demarginating intravascular neutrophils.

95

TABLE 6.2

Management of active ileocecal Crohn's disease

General measures

Explanation, psychosocial support
- physicians, specialist nurses
- patient support groups

Specialist multidisciplinary care
- physicians, surgeons, nutritionists, nurses, counselor

Establishing the diagnosis, site, extent and severity

Clinical evaluation
- complete blood cell count, ESR, C-reactive protein, ferritin, folate, B_{12}, albumin, liver-function tests, calcium, magnesium, zinc
- stool microscopy, culture, *C. difficile* toxin
- plain abdominal X-ray
- consider colonoscopy and biopsy, small-bowel barium radiology, ultrasound, CT scan, MRI, leukocyte scan

Monitoring progress

Daily clinical assessment

Stool chart

4-hourly temperature, pulse

Alternate daily complete blood cell count, ESR, C-reactive protein, urea and electrolytes, albumin

Daily plain abdominal X-ray (in patients with obstruction)

Supportive treatment

Fluids, electrolytes (sodium, potassium), blood transfusion

Nutritional supplementation; low-residue diet if small-bowel strictures

Subcutaneous heparin

Hematinics (B_{12}, folate)

Analgesia, antidiarrheals

Avoid NSAIDs, delayed-release drugs

(CONTINUED)

TABLE 6.2 (CONTINUED)

Specific treatments (separately or in combination)

Medical

- intravenous (hydrocortisone or methylprednisolone) then oral corticosteroids (prednisolone or budesonide)
- continue high-dose mesalazine in patients already taking it; otherwise consider starting when improvement begins
- consider metronidazole, ciprofloxacin, clarithromycin
- consider azathioprine/6-MP (slow responders) or infliximab for steroid non-responders

Nutritional

- liquid formula diet

Surgical

- resection or stricturoplasty

CT, computed tomography; ESR, erythrocyte sedimentation rate; 6-MP, 6-mercaptopurine; MRI, magnetic resonance imaging; NSAID, non-steroidal anti-inflammatory drug.

Endoscopy and biopsy. In patients with right iliac fossa pain where the diagnosis of Crohn's disease is in doubt, colonoscopy to the terminal ileum, with appropriate biopsies, can be helpful. It can also be used to balloon-dilate short strictures (see below). In established Crohn's colitis, colonoscopy during acute relapse is not routinely necessary and may be unsafe, as in active ulcerative colitis (Chapter 5). In previously undiagnosed patients, digital rectal examination and cautious sigmoidoscopy may show rectal induration or ulceration, or the presence of perianal disease. Furthermore, biopsies of macroscopically normal rectal mucosa may reveal epithelioid granulomas in a minority of patients with more proximal Crohn's disease.

Plain abdominal X-ray. A plain film is essential if intestinal obstruction is suspected. It may also show a mass in the right iliac fossa and, in active Crohn's colitis, provide information about disease extent and severity.

Barium radiology. Because it may exacerbate obstructive symptoms and pre-existing perforation, conventional barium follow through and small-bowel enema should be avoided in severely ill patients with small-bowel disease; CT scanning is a better alternative (see below). Contrast fistulography is useful in patients with abdominal sinuses or fistulas.

Radiolabeled leukocyte scans. ^{99}Tc-HMPAO scanning can help to identify, non-invasively, not only sites of intestinal inflammation, as in ulcerative colitis, but also intra-abdominal abscesses in patients with fever and/or an abdominal mass (see Chapter 3).

Ultrasound, CT scan and MRI. Abdominal ultrasound and a CT scan can be very useful in active Crohn's disease for the evaluation and percutaneous drainage of localized collections (see Chapter 3). Endoluminal ultrasound and MRI (Figure 6.1) are useful for the anatomic delineation of perianal abscesses and fistulas.

Supportive treatment. Patients with active Crohn's disease, like those with acute severe ulcerative colitis, need meticulous supportive treatment, including as necessary:
• intravenous fluids and electrolytes
• blood transfusion
• prophylactic subcutaneous heparin.

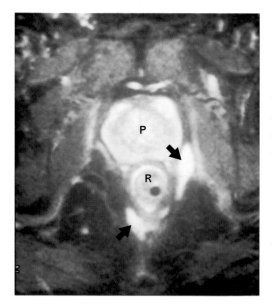

Figure 6.1 MRI showing a high-intensity signal track (arrowed) in a patient with Crohn's disease, indicating a posterior perianal collection with a fistulous track extending into the left ischiorectal fossa.
P, prostate; R, rectum.
Reproduced courtesy of Dr A McLean, Barts and The London NHS Trust, London, UK.

General nutritional and dietary measures, drug therapy and drugs to avoid are outlined in Table 6.2.

Active ileocecal Crohn's disease

Therapeutic options include drugs, a liquid formula diet and surgery (see Chapter 7), as separate alternatives or in combination, depending on the patient's age, presentation and personal preference (Table 6.2).

Drug therapy

Corticosteroids. In active disease, oral steroids provide the quickest and most reliable response (60–80% of patients). Conventionally, prednisolone, 40–60 mg/day, is used, the dose being tapered by 5 mg every 7–10 days once improvement has begun, usually after 3–4 weeks. Very sick patients or those needing to fast because of intestinal obstruction need intravenous corticosteroids at least initially (e.g. hydrocortisone, 300–400 mg/day; methylprednisolone, 40–60 mg/day). In patients able to take oral treatment in whom systemic steroid side effects are a major problem, budesonide (controlled ileal release, 9 mg/day) can be used, albeit at greater financial cost.

Up to 20% of patients with Crohn's disease may be difficult to wean off steroids after relapse. Of these, many will be able partially or totally to discontinue steroid therapy on the introduction of an aminosalicylate or immunomodulatory agent (see below), but a few will need to take oral prednisolone in the long term, with a consequent risk of side effects.

Aminosalicylates. Patients with only moderately active ileocecal disease, most of whom can be managed as outpatients, can be tried on high-dose oral mesalazine; about 40% will go into remission in 2–3 months. This treatment may be preferred by individuals who are reluctant to use corticosteroids.

Metronidazole and ciprofloxacin are modestly effective in mild to moderately active colonic Crohn's disease, but they are insufficiently potent for use as sole therapy in patients who are ill enough to need admission. Preliminary reports of the efficacy of clarithromycin and rifabutin, alone or in combination, need confirmation.

Immunosuppressive drugs. Patients who do not respond to corticosteroids, or relapse on their withdrawal, and who need to avoid operative treatment if possible because of extensive disease or previous surgery, can be treated with adjunctive oral azathioprine, 2.0–2.5 mg/kg/day, or 6-MP, 1.0–1.5 mg/kg/day, the dose of steroids being reduced and/or phased out altogether as remission is achieved. Such patients must be well enough to wait for up to 4 months for this to occur. The side effects of azathioprine and 6-MP make frequent blood counts and liver-function tests mandatory (see Chapter 4 and Table 4.4).

Azathioprine and 6-MP are long-term options for Crohn's disease. However, in patients maintained in full remission on azathioprine or 6-MP, the risk of relapse after 4 years of treatment appears to be similar whether the drug is continued or stopped. In view of the potential toxicity associated with long-term use of these drugs, their withdrawal should be considered in patients who are still in remission after 4 years of treatment.

Methotrexate is effective in about 40% of patients with steroid-refractory Crohn's disease when given intramuscularly or orally once a week. Its use is usually reserved for patients who are unresponsive to, or intolerant of, thiopurines, and it requires appropriate monitoring (see Chapter 4).

Infliximab, an anti-TNFα antibody, is available for use in patients with Crohn's disease refractory to steroids and/or conventional immunomodulatory drugs, and in whom surgery is inappropriate (see Chapter 4, Table 4.6). In this group, a single infusion of infliximab produces improvement by 4 weeks in most patients, and remission (CDAI < 150) in about a third. Patients tend to relapse in the ensuing 2–4 months, so repeated infusions at intervals of no more than 8–15 weeks, in conjunction with an immunomodulatory drug such as azathioprine, are often needed to maintain remission.

Dietary therapy. In patients with a poor response to corticosteroids, or a preference for avoiding them, in those with extensive small-bowel disease, and in children (see Chapter 8), a liquid formula diet is an alternative primary therapy. This can be either elemental (amino-acid-

based), oligomeric protein hydrolysate (containing peptides) or
polymeric protein (containing whole protein and not, therefore,
hypoallergenic), and is usually given for 4–6 weeks as the sole
nutritional source (Table 6.3).

TABLE 6.3

Entered nutrition in Crohn's disease

Preparations	Elemental
	Oligomeric
	Polymeric
Indications	Active small-bowel Crohn's disease
	Undernutrition in IBD
Side effects	
Intolerance	Taste, boredom, nasogastric tube, nausea
Diarrhea	Concurrent antibiotics, hyperosmolality, too fast administration
Metabolic	Fluid overload or depletion, hypo- or hyperglycemia, low sodium/potassium/phosphate
Pulmonary aspiration	
Placement difficulties	
Monitoring	Fluid balance chart
	Twice-weekly weight, urea and electrolytes, glucose, albumin
Contraindications	Severe diarrhea
	Patient refusal
Mechanisms of action (all speculative)	Hypoallergenic
	Bowel rest
	Altered bacterial flora
	Reduced gut permeability
	Altered gut immunity
	Nutritional repletion (including essential micronutrients)

This approach is probably as effective as corticosteroid therapy in the short term, as about 60% of patients achieve remission. Unfortunately, after the resumption of a normal diet, many patients relapse (50% at 6 months). Whether this can be prevented by the selective and gradual reintroduction of particular low-fat, low-fiber foods to which individual patients are not intolerant, or by the intermittent use of further enteral feeding for short periods, remains to be proven.

The success of enteral nutrition as a primary therapy for Crohn's disease is also limited by:

- its cost
- the unpleasant taste of some of the available preparations
- the frequent need to give the feed by nasogastric tube
- poor compliance.

Nevertheless, such therapy does offer a valuable alternative in the well-motivated minority of adults for whom it is appropriate.

Surgery (limited right hemicolectomy) is indicated in the 20–40% of patients whose ileocecal disease fails to respond to drug or dietary therapy, particularly if they have short-segment (less than 200 mm) rather than extensive disease (see Chapter 7). Indeed, some patients prefer surgery to the prospect of pharmacological or nutritional treatment of uncertain duration. There are no controlled data to confirm which approach is best. After surgery, there is a 50% chance of recurrent symptoms at 5 years and of further surgery at 10 years; taking a long-term aminosalicylate and stopping smoking may reduce these risks by up to 50%.

Specific treatment of other presentations of active Crohn's disease

The general principles of the management of other presentations of active Crohn's disease are the same as those described above. Specific management aspects are outlined below.

Obstructive small-bowel Crohn's disease. In patients presenting with obstructive symptoms and signs (Chapter 2), and with corresponding abnormalities on plain abdominal X-ray (Figure 6.2), the principal difficulty lies in deciding whether stricturing is due to active inflammation, fibrosis with scarring or even adhesions. Sometimes laboratory markers (e.g. raised platelet count, ESR, C-reactive protein) and/or radiolabeled leukocyte scans can help to identify individuals with active inflammatory Crohn's disease, but in most instances a short trial of intravenous corticosteroids is given in addition to intravenous fluids and, if necessary, nasogastric suction (Table 6.4). Parenteral nutrition is required if resumption of an oral diet is not likely in 5–7 days.

If the stricture is in the upper jejunum, terminal ileum or colon, enteroscopic or colonoscopic balloon dilation can be undertaken (Figure 6.3). In patients who do not settle after 48–72 hours of conservative treatment, surgery is needed; the options are local resection or, for short and/or multiple strictures, stricturoplasty (see Chapter 7). Patients responding to conservative therapy should be advised to take a low-residue diet (see above) to reduce the chance of recurrent symptoms.

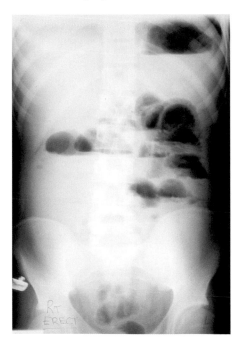

Figure 6.2 Plain abdominal X-ray showing small-bowel obstruction due to terminal ileal stricturing in Crohn's disease.

TABLE 6.4

Specific treatments for other presentations of active Crohn's disease*

Subacute obstruction	Trial of intravenous corticosteroids Intravenous fluids and nasogastric suction (if necessary) Surgery for non-responders: local resection or stricturoplasty
Intra-abdominal abscess	Broad-spectrum antibiotics Percutaneous or surgical drainage
Intestinal fistula	Enteral or parenteral nutrition Oral metronidazole (for up to 3 months) Oral azathioprine or 6-MP Consider intravenous infliximab Surgery: local resection
Perianal disease	Oral metronidazole (for up to 3 months), ciprofloxacin Oral azathioprine or 6-MP Consider intravenous infliximab or ciclosporin Surgery: drain abscesses, seton sutures for chronic fistulas
Oral and upper gastrointestinal disease	Treat as in other sites Oral, topical or intralesional corticosteroids Omeprazole for duodenal disease

*Presentations other than ileocecal disease (Table 6.2) or Crohn's colitis (Table 6.5).
6-MP, 6-mercaptopurine.

Intra-abdominal abscess. Ultrasound, CT and/or radiolabeled leukocyte scans are usually used to confirm the diagnosis of intra-abdominal abscess in Crohn's patients presenting with pain, weight loss, diarrhea and fever with or without a tender mass (Figure 6.4). Broad-spectrum antibiotics are given and the abscess drained either percutaneously under radiological control, and/or surgically (Table 6.4). When oral food intake is likely to be restricted for more than 5 days, parenteral nutrition should be started. Subsequent treatment is usually of the underlying pathological process, for example ileocecal inflammation.

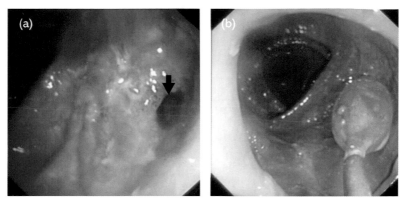

Figure 6.3 Colonoscopic balloon dilation of an anastomotic stricture in Crohn's disease: (a) narrowed ileocolonic anastomosis (arrowed); (b) through-the-scope balloon inserted into stricture and inflated.

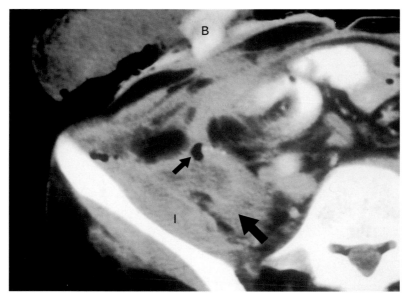

Figure 6.4 CT scan showing a psoas abscess in a patient with an ileostomy after total colectomy for Crohn's disease. Note the ileostomy bag (B) on the anterior abdominal wall with a short fistula (small arrow) leading from dilated prestomal small bowel into an abscess in psoas muscle (large arrow) adjacent to iliacus (I). Reproduced courtesy of Dr A McLean, Barts and The London NHS Trust, London, UK.

Intestinal fistula. The relevant anatomic connections are clarified using contrast radiology, CT scans, endoluminal ultrasound and/or MRI (see above, 'Establishing the diagnosis'). Nutritional well-being should be restored using enteral or parenteral nutrition (Table 6.4). Where there is no obstruction distal to the site of intestinal fistulas, medical therapy with oral, rectal or intravenous metronidazole and/or oral azathioprine or 6-MP will cause some fistulas to heal; repeated anti-TNFα antibody (infliximab) infusions (see below) are a newer option. All patients with enterourinary or enterovaginal fistulas, and most with enterocutaneous fistulas, however, require surgical resection of the fistula and local resection of involved intestine and/or other viscera (see Chapter 7).

Perianal disease. Non-suppurative perianal Crohn's disease may respond to oral metronidazole and/or ciprofloxacin given for up to 3 months, and to azathioprine or 6-MP in the long term (Table 6.4). Healing of more than 50% of perianal (and other) fistulas has been reported in about 60% of patients treated with intravenous infusions of infliximab; however, fistulas often reopen in the ensuing months. Patients with suppurating perianal Crohn's disease need surgery, minimized as far as possible (see Chapter 7). In severe perianal disease, however, radical surgery with proctocolectomy may eventually prove necessary.

Crohn's colitis. The treatment of active Crohn's colitis closely resembles that of active ulcerative colitis (Table 5.1); differences are outlined in Table 6.5. Unlike ulcerative colitis, moderately active Crohn's colitis may be improved by oral metronidazole, 400 mg twice daily for up to 3 months, if tolerated, in up to 50% of patients who wish to avoid corticosteroids or aminosalicylates. Liquid formula diets may also be effective, but Crohn's colitis responds less well than ileocecal disease to this form of therapy.

In patients who require total colectomy, permanent ileostomy is preferable to an ileoanal pouch because of the high incidence of pouch failure and sepsis in Crohn's disease (see Chapter 7). In rare individuals with refractory segmental colitis, local resection of short diseased segments can be performed.

TABLE 6.5

Specific treatment of active Crohn's colitis

Medical therapy	Corticosteroids, intravenous (hydrocortisone or methylprednisolone) then oral (prednisolone)
	5-ASA orally
	Metronidazole orally (for mild cases)
	Azathioprine/6-MP orally if response can be postponed for up to 4 months
	Infliximab for non-responders
Nutritional therapy	Liquid formula diet
Surgery	Total colectomy with ileostomy (ileoanal pouch contraindicated)
	Segmental resection for stricture

5-ASA, 5-aminosalicylate; 6-MP, 6-mercaptopurine.

Toxic megacolon is even more rare in acute severe Crohn's than it is in ulcerative colitis.

Oral and upper gastrointestinal Crohn's disease. Treatment of oral and upper gastrointestinal Crohn's disease follows the usual principles outlined above. Patients with oral Crohn's disease are best managed in close conjunction with specialists in oral medicine. Particular treatment options include topical and intralesional steroids and topical tacrolimus paste; some food constituents should be avoided (e.g. benzoate and cinnamon). Duodenal Crohn's disease may respond to omeprazole; endoscopic balloon dilation of strictures can also be helpful, but surgery may be technically demanding and complicated by fistulation.

Maintaining remission

The most effective prophylactic measure in patients who smoke is to stop: the risk of relapse in non-smokers at 5 years is reduced by about 30%. The efficacy of drug prophylaxis depends on whether remission has been achieved by medical or surgical treatment.

Strategies for maintaining remission are listed in Table 6.6.

TABLE 6.6

Maintenance of remission in Crohn's disease

All patients	Stop smoking
Remission achieved by medical treatment	No standard treatment of proven value
	Azathioprine/6-MP or methotrexate for refractory Crohn's disease
	Fish oil (possibly)
Remission achieved by surgery	Aminosalicylates (small-bowel disease only)
	Metronidazole (3 months only)
	Budesonide (for active not fibrostenotic Crohn's disease)

6-MP, 6-mercaptopurine.

Patients in remission after medical treatment. Meta-analysis shows that, unlike in ulcerative colitis, long-term aminosalicylates have little or no prophylactic effect in this setting. Prednisolone has no routine prophylactic role, not least because of its side effects. Unfortunately, budesonide, 6 mg/day, although less likely to cause steroid-related complications such as osteoporosis, does not reduce the relapse rate at 1 year. In the minority of patients who depend on long-term corticosteroids and in whom symptoms recur whenever the dose is reduced, azathioprine, 6-MP and methotrexate are of proven value in maintaining remission and reducing steroid requirements. High-potency ileal-release fish-oil capsules, if commercially available, would be an attractive option should the prophylactic efficacy reported in one study be confirmed.

Patients in remission after surgical treatment. After resection for ileocecal disease, there is a 50% chance of recurrence needing further surgery at 10 years. In patients with exclusively small-bowel disease, long-term aminosalicylates reduce the risk of symptomatic relapse after resection by about 50%, but the best dose and preparation are uncertain; limited data suggest that at least 3 g/day of mesalazine should be used. In patients with colonic Crohn's disease, aminosalicylates have no preventive role postoperatively. Budesonide,

6 mg/day, reduces the endoscopic recurrence rate by 50% at 1 year for active, but not fibrostenotic, Crohn's disease. Oral metronidazole, 400 mg three times daily for 3 months postoperatively, reduces the symptomatic relapse rate at 1 year, but not beyond this period. Limited data suggest that thiopurines may have a prophylactic role after surgery, but confirmation is required before evidence-based recommendations can be made.

Follow-up. The rarity with which primary care physicians see patients with Crohn's disease, and the wide variety of its manifestations and complications, mean that most patients should be followed up in specialist hospital clinics (Table 5.1).

Patients with active disease or those receiving therapy need more frequent hospital review for:
- adjustment of their treatment according to the progress of their disease
- monitoring of side effects (see Tables 4.1, 4.3 and 4.4).

For patients in remission and receiving no therapy, follow-up may take place at annual intervals, and may need to include tests to check for:
- occult disease activity (blood count, ESR, C-reactive protein, albumin, fecal calprotectin levels)
- undernutrition (weight, body mass index; serum albumin, calcium, phosphate and sometimes magnesium and zinc; red-cell folate; serum vitamin B_{12} levels in patients with terminal ileal disease or resection)
- osteoporosis (bone densitometry)
- other complications of Crohn's disease, such as liver disease (liver-function tests).

Although the risk of colorectal cancer is increased in patients with Crohn's colitis, particularly if it is extensive, the place of screening for colorectal cancer in Crohn's disease is even more uncertain than in ulcerative colitis, and few centers offer routine colonoscopic surveillance of asymptomatic patients for this purpose.

Key points – medical management of Crohn's disease

- The treatment of active Crohn's disease depends on its site and the nature of the pathological process causing the patient's symptoms.
- Therapeutic options for active Crohn's disease include corticosteroids, aminosalicylates, antibiotics, a liquid formula diet, immunomodulatory agents, surgery and infliximab.
- All patients with Crohn's disease should be encouraged to stop smoking, given the adverse effect of smoking on the natural history of the disease.
- Patients with Crohn's disease should participate in decisions about their treatment, particularly in relation to the use of new biological therapies or possible surgery.

Key references

Cammá C, Giunta M, Rosselli M et al. Mesalazine in the maintenance treatment of Crohn's disease: a meta-analysis adjusted for confounding variables. *Gastroenterology* 1997;113:1465–73.

Griffiths AM, Ohlsson A, Scherman PM et al. Meta-analysis of enteral nutrition as a primary treatment of active Crohn's disease. *Gastroenterology* 1995;108:1056–67.

Hanauer SB, Feagan BG, Lichtenstein GR et al. Maintenance infliximab for Crohn's disease: the ACCENT 1 randomised trial. *Lancet* 2002;359: 1541–9.

Hanauer SB, Sandborn W. Management of Crohn's disease in adults. *Am J Gastroenterol* 2001; 96:635–43.

Papi C, Luchetti R, Gili L et al. Budesonide in the treatment of Crohn's disease: a meta-analysis. *Aliment Pharmacol Ther* 2000; 14:1419–28.

Pearson DC, May GR, Fick GH et al. Azathioprine and 6-mercaptopurine in Crohn's disease: a meta-analysis. *Ann Intern Med* 1995;122:132–42.

Sands BE, Anderson FH, Bernstein CN et al. Infliximab maintenance therapy for fistulizing Crohn's disease. *N Engl J Med* 2004;350: 934–6.

Summers RW, Switz DM, Sessions JT et al. National co-operative Crohn's disease study: results of drug treatment. *Gastroenterology* 1979; 77:847–69.

The management of both ulcerative colitis and Crohn's disease requires close liaison between physician and surgeon. Specialist nursing care, including that from a stoma therapist, is also necessary both pre- and postoperatively. Dieticians and counselors may also play a key role in preparing patients physically and mentally for surgery and its consequences.

Ulcerative colitis

Indications for surgery (Table 7.1) are as follows.

Emergency colectomy, after appropriate immediate resuscitation (see Chapter 5), is necessary in patients with colonic perforation or massive hemorrhage.

TABLE 7.1

Surgery in ulcerative colitis

Indication	
Emergency	Colonic perforation
	Massive colonic hemorrhage
Urgent	Deterioration or non-response to medical treatment of acute severe ulcerative colitis in 5–8 days
	Toxic megacolon
Elective	Chronic active (steroid-dependent or refractory) ulcerative colitis
	Dysplasia in cancer
	Refractory pyoderma gangrenosum (rarely)
	Growth retardation in children (rarely)
Options	Restorative proctocolectomy with ileoanal pouch
	Proctocolectomy with ileostomy
	Colectomy with ileorectal anastomosis

Urgent colectomy is needed in patients with acute severe ulcerative colitis who deteriorate, fail to respond to intensive medical treatment in 5–8 days or develop toxic colonic dilation that does not respond within 24 hours to more intense medical treatment (Chapter 5).

Elective colectomy is indicated in refractory, often steroid-dependent chronic active ulcerative colitis, and dysplasia or frank carcinoma (Chapter 5). Occasionally, elective colectomy may be necessary in children with chronically active disease to prevent growth retardation (Chapter 8) and, very rarely, in patients with intractable extraintestinal complications dependent on colonic disease activity, such as pyoderma gangrenosum.

Options for surgery are outlined below, and summarized in Table 7.1 and Figure 7.1.

Proctocolectomy with permanent ileostomy has the lowest morbidity and mortality of the available surgical options, is technically the easiest, and involves only one operation.

Colectomy with ileorectal anastomosis is useful for older patients with relative rectal sparing who could not cope with a stoma or are

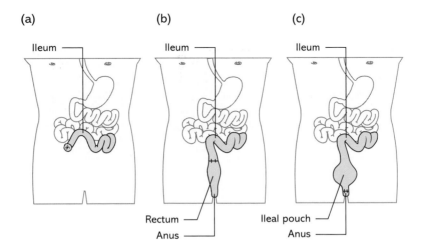

(a)   **(b)**   **(c)**

Ileum   Ileum   Ileum

Rectum   Ileal pouch

Anus   Anus

Figure 7.1 Surgical options in ulcerative colitis: (a) panproctocolectomy with ileostomy; (b) subtotal colectomy with ileorectal anastomosis; (c) total colectomy with ileoanal pouch.

unsuitable for an ileoanal pouch because of physical frailty or poor anal sphincter function. It is contraindicated in any patient with pronounced rectal inflammation (since they will continue to have bleeding, diarrhea and urgency postoperatively), and in young patients (in view of the long-term risk of cancer developing in the retained rectum, for which annual sigmoidoscopy with biopsies for dysplasia would be necessary indefinitely; see Chapter 5).

Restorative proctocolectomy with ileoanal pouch is the most recently devised procedure for ulcerative colitis, and avoids the need for permanent ileostomy. It is now the favored operation in younger patients (usually younger than 60 years) in whom preoperative confirmation of normal anal sphincter function minimizes the risk of postoperative incontinence of liquid pouch contents. The operation to fashion an ileoanal reservoir ('pouch') is technically difficult, and usually requires a temporary loop ileostomy that is closed at a second operation a few months later.

Complications of the different surgical options are as follows.

Ileostomy. Although proctocolectomy and ileostomy have the lowest morbidity and mortality of operations for ulcerative colitis, ileostomy incurs a readmission rate of about 50% in 10 years. Complications are listed in Table 7.2: specialist stoma therapists are crucial for their management.

Ileoanal pouch. Complications of ileoanal pouch surgery (Table 7.3) lead to excision of the pouch and conversion to permanent ileostomy ('pouch failure') in about 10% of patients. Early pouch failure is so common in patients with Crohn's colitis that formation of an ileoanal pouch is contraindicated after colectomy for Crohn's disease or indeterminate colitis (see below). Even in patients judged to have had successful pouch surgery, daytime stool frequency is four to seven, urgency is common and nocturnal incontinence is present in about 20% of patients.

Pouchitis. Villous atrophy and colonic metaplasia occur normally in ileoanal pouches. The diagnosis of pouchitis is made in patients with worsening diarrhea, endoscopic signs of inflammation and

TABLE 7.2

Complications of ileostomy

Complication	Comment
Early	
Skin problems	Rare now with stoma therapists and improved appliances
Adhesive intestinal obstruction	May need surgery
Necrosis, fistulas, retraction, parasternal herniation	Requires refashioning of stoma
Excess stomal output (normal approximately 500 mL/day)	Improves with time postoperatively; avoid salt depletion in hot weather
Late	
Sexual dysfunction	Due to psychogenic factors or surgical pelvic nerve damage
Uric acid renal stones	Due to excess alkaline stomal output

histological evidence of acute inflammation with neutrophil infiltration and ulceration. Its etiology is unknown: it may represent recurrent ulcerative colitis in the pouch, or it may be a consequence of ischemia, changes in bacterial flora, or mucosal damage induced by bile salts. About 40% of patients will have at least one episode in the first 10 years after pouch construction. Therapeutic options include metronidazole, 400–800 mg twice daily for 10 days, and topical or oral corticosteroids or aminosalicylates (as for ulcerative colitis; see Tables 4.2 and 4.3). Recent controlled data suggest that probiotic treatment with VSL3, a sachet containing a cocktail of bifidobacteria, lactobacilli and streptococci, is an effective therapy for pouchitis. However, a minority of patients with refractory pouchitis require pouch resection and a permanent ileostomy.

TABLE 7.3

Complications of ileoanal pouch

Complication	Comment
Early	
Pelvic sepsis	Needs antibiotics, drainage and/or surgery
Anastomotic leaks	Needs pouch tube drainage and sometimes surgery
Adhesive intestinal obstruction	May need surgery
Late	
Poor function	Excessive diarrhea, urgency, incontinence
Sexual dysfunction	Due to psychogenic factors or surgical pelvic nerve damage
Pouchitis	See page 113
Vitamin B_{12} deficiency	Treat with intramuscular hydroxocobalamin
Pouch failure	Needs conversion to ileostomy (in 10% of patients)

Crohn's disease

Indications. Surgery is indicated primarily for disease refractory to medical and/or nutritional therapy, or for complications (Table 7.4). In Crohn's disease, unlike ulcerative colitis, surgery is not curative: recurrence at the surgical anastomosis or elsewhere in the gastrointestinal tract is common.

Options. The major principle of surgery for Crohn's disease is to conserve as much bowel as possible; excision of the minimum amount of bowel necessary to remove macroscopic disease is recommended.

In some centers, operations for Crohn's disease are now performed laparoscopically.

TABLE 7.4

Surgery in Crohn's disease

Indications

Emergency	Free perforation (rare)
	Massive hemorrhage (rare)
Urgent/soon	Small-bowel obstruction
	Small-bowel inflammation refractory to medical treatment
	Crohn's colitis
	Intra-abdominal abscess
	Enterocutaneous, -urinary or -vaginal fistulas
	Perianal abscess
	Toxic megacolon (rare)
	Carcinoma (rare)

Options

Small-bowel disease	Local resection
	Stricturoplasty
Terminal ileal disease	Right hemicolectomy
Colitis	Proctocolectomy with ileostomy
	Colectomy with ileorectal anastomosis (rarely)
	Segmental resection for localized disease (rarely)
Perianal disease	Lay open complex fistulas, drain with seton sutures
	Drain abscesses
	Proctocolectomy (rarely)

Small-bowel or ileal resection. Discrete segments of small bowel are removed with an end-to-end anastomosis. Ileocecal disease is excised with a limited right hemicolectomy, in which the ileum is anastomosed to the ascending colon, with removal of involved ileum, cecum and appendix.

Stricturoplasty. In patients with obstructive symptoms due to very short and/or multiple strictured segments of small-bowel Crohn's disease, the risk of short bowel syndrome (see Chapter 2) following

(a)   (b)

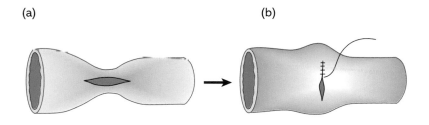

Figure 7.2 Stricturoplasty for Crohn's disease: (a) longitudinal incision through stricture; (b) incision sewn up transversely to widen lumen.

excision can be averted by stricturoplasty, in which a longitudinal incision of the stricture is sewn up transversely, with consequent widening of the gut lumen (Figure 7.2).

Surgery for colonic Crohn's disease. For patients with extensive Crohn's colitis refractory to medical therapy, the safest operation is proctocolectomy with ileostomy (Figure 7.1). Ileoanal pouch creation is contraindicated by a high frequency of anastomotic leaks and sepsis, which necessitate its removal. Even in patients with rectal sparing, the recurrence rate is much higher with colectomy and ileorectal anastomosis than with proctocolectomy and ileostomy, making the latter preferable. In rare patients with very localized colonic disease, segmental resection (unlike in ulcerative colitis) is a reasonable option.

Surgery for perianal disease. As in other sites of Crohn's disease, surgery should be minimized, not least because of the risks of inducing incontinence as a result of iatrogenic sphincter damage. Abscesses require drainage and complex chronic fistulas may need insertion of loose (seton) sutures to facilitate continued drainage. Defunctioning ileostomy or colostomy may allow healing of severe perianal disease by diverting the fecal stream, but recurrence after closure of the stoma is common. Strictures can be treated with cautious dilation (to avoid sphincter damage). The threshold for biopsy should be low in view of the occasional development of anal carcinoma in relation to chronic perianal Crohn's disease. Proctectomy is sometimes needed for severe and refractory anorectal Crohn's disease.

TABLE 7.5

Long-term complications of resection for ileocecal Crohn's disease

Recurrence of Crohn's disease

Bile-salt malabsorption
- Cholegenic diarrhea
- Enteric hyperoxaluria, urinary oxalate stones
- Gallstones

Vitamin B_{12} deficiency

Complications of removing the terminal ileum for ileocecal or ileal Crohn's disease (right hemicolectomy) are summarized below and in Table 7.5.

Recurrence of Crohn's disease. In about 70% of patients, colonoscopy shows recurrent aphthoid ulceration, usually immediately proximal to the anastomosis, 1 year after right hemicolectomy. Long-term oral aminosalicylates or postoperative treatment with oral metronidazole for 3 months reduces the endoscopic recurrence rate at 1 year, but the effect of such therapy on the symptomatic recurrence rate of 50% at 5 years and the rate of need for repeat surgery of 50% at 10 years is not clear (see Chapter 6). Stopping smoking reduces the recurrence rate.

Bile-salt malabsorption. By removing their site of absorption, terminal ileal resection leads to the passage of primary bile salts (cholate and chenodeoxycholate) into the colon, where they:
- induce mucosal secretion of water and electrolytes (with resultant diarrhea)
- increase mucosal permeability to dietary oxalate (predisposing to enteric hyperoxaluria and urinary oxalate stones)
- cause fecal loss of bile salts (increasing the risk of cholesterol gallstones).

As intestinal adaptation occurs postoperatively, cholegenic diarrhea often improves; in the interim, symptomatic treatment with antidiarrheal agents, such as codeine phosphate or loperamide, or with a bile-salt-binding ion-exchange resin, such as colestyramine (cholestyramine), may help.

Enteric hyperoxaluria is treated with a low oxalate (i.e. avoiding spinach, rhubarb, beetroot, strawberries, chocolate, tea, coffee, cola), low-fat, high-calcium, high-fluid diet.

Vitamin B_{12} deficiency. After surgery involving terminal ileal resection, particularly if more than 1000 mm has been removed, patients should have annual checks of their serum vitamin B_{12} level, with replacement by hydroxocobalamin, 1000 µg intramuscularly every 3 months, in the event of deficiency.

Key points – surgery

- Surgery offers a cure for ulcerative colitis, but there is always a risk of recurrence of Crohn's disease after resection.
- The patient should be closely involved in the decision to undertake surgery.

Key references

Delaney CP, Fazio VW. Crohn's disease of the small bowel. *Surg Clin N Am* 2001;81:137–58.

Gionchetti P, Rizzello F, Venturi A et al. Oral bacteriotherapy as maintenance treatment in patients with chronic pouchitis: a double-blind, placebo-controlled trial. *Gastroenterology* 2000;119:305–9.

Lee ECG, Papaioannou N. Minimal surgery for chronic obstruction in patients with extensive or universal Crohn's disease. *Ann R Coll Surg Engl* 1982;64:229–33.

Stocchi L, Pemberton JH. Pouch and pouchitis. *Gastroenterol Clin N Am* 2001;30:223–41.

Fertility

Female fertility is not impaired except in active IBD. Because of the risk of inadequate absorption, women with diarrhea due to IBD should not rely exclusively on the oral contraceptive pill to prevent pregnancy.

In male patients taking sulfasalazine, fertility is reduced as a result of azoospermia, but this can be reversed within a few weeks by switching to an alternative aminosalicylate (see Tables 4.2 and 4.3).

Pregnancy and lactation

Outcome of pregnancy is normal in patients with quiescent IBD, but there is an increased rate of spontaneous abortion, premature delivery and stillbirth in those with persistently active disease.

Activity of IBD. Pregnancy itself has no consistent effect on the activity of IBD, although the disease occasionally flares early in the puerperium.

Treatment. Corticosteroids and aminosalicylates can be used safely during pregnancy and lactation; withholding them exposes the mother and fetus unnecessarily to the adverse consequences of active disease. Azathioprine and 6-MP should be avoided during pregnancy if possible because of their teratogenic potential. However, accidental pregnancies in patients taking azathioprine have been uneventful. Other immunomodulatory drugs and prolonged courses of metronidazole are contraindicated in pregnancy. Although currently contraindicated in pregnancy, inadvertent use of infliximab in this setting has not been associated with an adverse outcome. Surgery is occasionally necessary in very sick patients, and is associated with a high rate of fetal loss.

IBD in childhood

Prevalence. Ulcerative colitis may occur at any age. Allergy to cows'-milk protein produces a similar syndrome in babies after weaning and needs to be excluded. Crohn's disease is rare in children under the age of 8, but its incidence in this age group appears to be increasing.

Diagnosis. The diagnosis of IBD in children is often delayed. It should be considered early in patients not only with classical symptoms, such as pain and diarrhea (see Chapter 2), but also in those with delayed growth and puberty. Prompt referral to a specialist pediatric gastroenterology unit is advised for appropriate investigation along conventional lines (see Chapter 3).

Treatment. The principles of treatment for children are the same as for adults. However, the adverse effects of IBD on growth and pubertal development mean that active disease should be suppressed as soon as possible, undernutrition reversed and prolonged courses of corticosteroids avoided. In pediatric and adolescent Crohn's disease, unlike in the adult disease, enteral nutrition with a liquid formula diet, given if necessary by fine-bore nasogastric tube (see page 102), plays a primary therapeutic role. Because of the need to maintain growth and development, prepubertal colectomy for ulcerative colitis and resection for Crohn's disease are also more frequently used than in adults. Azathioprine is a useful option in steroid-dependent children in whom surgery is inappropriate or declined. In all children with IBD, growth should be carefully monitored on weight-for-height charts.

Key points – IBD in pregnancy and childhood

- Most patients with IBD have uneventful pregnancies, provided they seek prompt treatment for relapses.
- Corticosteroids, aminosalicylates and azathioprine appear to be well tolerated in pregnancy, but some gastroenterologists recommend that azathioprine be avoided in planned pregnancies because of its potential teratogenicity.
- To maximize growth in children, active IBD should be promptly suppressed and prolonged courses of corticosteroids avoided.
- A liquid formula diet is the preferred first-line treatment in children with active Crohn's disease.

Key references

Barton JR, Ferguson A. Clinical features, morbidity and mortality of Scottish children with inflammatory bowel disease. *Q J Med* 1990;75: 423–39.

Connell W, Miller A. Treating inflammatory bowel disease during pregnancy: risks and safety of drug therapy. *Drug Saf* 1999;21:311–23.

Dejaco C, Mittermaier C, Reinisch W et al. Azathioprine treatment and male fertility in inflammatory bowel disease. *Gastroenterology* 2001;121: 1048–53.

Diav-Citrin O, Park YH, Veersuntharam G et al. The safety of mesalamine in human pregnancy: a prospective controlled cohort study. *Gastroenterology* 1998;114:23–8.

Escher JC, Taminiau JAJM, Nieuwenhuis EES et al. Treatment of inflammatory bowel disease in childhood: best available evidence. *Inflamm Bowel Dis* 2003;9:34–58.

Heuschkel RB, Walker-Smith JA. Enteral nutrition in inflammatory bowel disease of childhood. *J Parenter Enteral Nutr* 1999;23: S29–32.

Hudson M, Flett G, Sinclair TS et al. Fertility and pregnancy in inflammatory bowel disease. *Int J Gynaecol Obstet* 1997;58:229–37.

Markowitz J, Grancher K, Kohn N et al. A multicenter trial of 6-mercaptopurine and prednisone in children with newly diagnosed Crohn's disease. *Gastroenterology* 2000;119:895–902.

Miller JP. Inflammatory bowel disease in pregnancy: a review. *J R Soc Med* 1986;79:2212–19.

Narendranathan M, Sandler RS, Suchindran M, et al. Male infertility in inflammatory bowel disease. *J Clin Gastroenterol* 1989;11:403–6.

Ulcerative colitis

Mortality. The risk of death in ulcerative colitis is highest in the first year of diagnosis and relates mainly to first attacks of acute severe ulcerative colitis. In this setting, it is now less than 2%, principal causes of death being pulmonary embolism, perforation and sepsis. The overall mortality of patients with ulcerative colitis is no different from that of the normal population, the risks of ulcerative colitis and associated colorectal cancer possibly being counterbalanced by the non-smoking status of most patients with the disease (see Chapter 1).

Morbidity. Most patients experience a relapsing and remitting course of disease; 70% of untreated patients have flare-ups annually. In patients with distal disease at presentation, extension to involve the proximal colon occurs in about 20% after 10 years. The cumulative colectomy rate in patients with total colitis is about 30% at 15 years.

Cancer risk. The risk of colorectal cancer is increased in patients who have had subtotal or total ulcerative colitis for more than 10 years, the cumulative risk being about 20% at 30 years. The prognosis of colonic cancer complicating ulcerative colitis resembles that of patients without colitis. Colonoscopic surveillance programs are widely used (see Chapter 5), but have not been proved to reduce mortality from colonic cancer in ulcerative colitis.

Crohn's disease

Mortality. The cumulative mortality of Crohn's disease is approximately twice that in the general population. Death is due predominantly to sepsis, pulmonary embolism, and complications of surgery and immunosuppressive therapy in patients with severe chronic disease.

Morbidity. A higher proportion of patients with Crohn's disease than with ulcerative colitis show a chronic active rather than a relapsing remitting course of disease. Surgery is required in about 50% of patients in the first 10 years after diagnosis. Of those having an operation, 50% will need further surgery in the next 10 years, the risks being higher in patients with ileal and ileocolonic disease than in those with purely colonic disease.

Key points – prognosis

- Mortality in ulcerative colitis resembles that in the general population, but in Crohn's disease it is increased twofold.
- Causes of death in patients with severe IBD include sepsis, pulmonary embolism, surgery and immunosuppressive therapy.
- The prevalence, chronicity and onset in early life of IBD mean that it represents a substantial burden of sickness both in the community and for healthcare resources.

Key references

Binder V, Hendriken C, Kreiner S. Prognosis in Crohn's disease – based on results from a regional patient group from the county of Copenhagen. *Gut* 1985;26:146–50.

Ekbom A, Helmick CG, Zack M et al. Survival and causes of death in patients with inflammatory bowel disease: a population-based study. *Gastroenterology* 1992;103:954–60.

Jess T, Winther KV, Munkholm P et al. Mortality and causes of death in Crohn's disease: follow up of a population-based cohort in Copenhagen County, Denmark. *Gastroenterology* 2002;122: 1808–14.

Langholz E, Munkholm P, Davidsen E, Binder V. Course of ulcerative colitis: analysis of changes in disease activity over years. *Gastroenterology* 1994;107:3–11.

Munkholm P, Langholz E, Davidsen E, Binder V. Intestinal cancer risk and mortality in patients with Crohn's disease. *Gastroenterology* 1993;105: 1716–23.

Genetics

The intense research effort under way to clarify the genetics of IBD is likely to have a major impact on its management in the near future. Identification of the genes involved, and the proteins they encode, will shed new light on the pathogenesis of the disease, and is likely to lead to new treatments. Such information will enable us to identify relatives of index patients who are at risk of developing IBD, to facilitate diagnosis, and to predict the phenotype and particularly the natural history of the disease in affected individuals. Advances in molecular biology are also likely to enable us to identify patients with IBD who are at particular risk of developing colorectal cancer; colonoscopic screening will become obsolete.

Diagnosis

Less invasive investigative techniques are imminent. Virtual colonoscopy is already available in some centers. MRI is likely to play an increasing role in the diagnosis and monitoring of complications of Crohn's disease, while positron emission tomography may become a useful way of assessing disease site and activity. Serological methods may soon allow the diagnosis of IBD in patients with ill-defined symptoms.

Therapy

Improvements in future medical treatments will take several directions. First, conventional therapies, such as steroids and aminosalicylates, will become available in formulations that focus delivery more accurately on the site of disease, thereby further reducing systemic side effects. More excitingly, a continuing increase in our knowledge of the etiology and pathogenesis of IBD will inevitably lead to the development of more selectively targeted therapies. Probiotic and prebiotic treatments may emerge from an appreciation of the importance of the intestinal flora in driving mucosal inflammation. Such treatments will be particularly useful for the maintenance of remission. Cytokine-based therapies, derived from progressive elucidation of the complexities of the inflammatory process, will undoubtedly follow infliximab into the therapeutic arena for patients with active disease; cytokine-based gene therapy, applied topically to affected gut mucosa, may prove an important step forward in ulcerative colitis and Crohn's disease, as in other chronic inflammatory diseases outside the gut. The choice of treatment in individual patients with IBD will depend, increasingly, not only on the phenotypic expression of their disease, but also on their genotype.

Teamwork

Whatever advances are made in the coming years, the management of patients with IBD will continue to require close collaboration between physicians, surgeons, specialist nurses, dieticians and counselors. In addition, a clinical geneticist may need to join this team. Most importantly, the patient with IBD must be looked upon as a person rather than a case. As management becomes more complex and the options more varied, it is essential that the patient remains at the center of the decision-making process. The individual with IBD must be the final arbiter of the type of therapy he or she is to be given.

Useful resources

Patient support groups

Australia
Australian Crohn's and Colitis
  Association
PO Box 201
Moorolbark
VIC 31 38
Tel: +61 (0)9726 9008
www.acca.net.au

Austria
Österreichische Morbus
  Crohn/Colitis Ulcerosa-
  Vereinigung (ÖMCCV)
Obere Augartenstraße 26–28
1020 Wien
Tel/fax: +43 (0)1 333 06 33
crohn-colitis@oemccv.or.at
www.oemccv.or.at/crohn-colitis

Belgium
Crohn En Colitis Ulcerosa
  Vereniging (CCV) vzw
Kapucijnenvoer 10
3000 Leuven
Tel: +32 (0)16 20 73 12
Fax: +32 (0)16 20 87 32
Tel/fax (secretariat):
+32 (0)16 56 83 69
secretariaat@ccv-vzw.be
www.ccv-vzw.be

Canada
Crohn's and Colitis Foundation
  of Canada
60 St Clair Avenue East
Suite 600
Toronto, ON M4T 1N5
Tel: +1 416 920 5035 /
  1 800 387 1479
Fax: +1 416 929 0364
ccfc@ccfc.ca
www.ccfc.ca

Czech Republic
CROCODILE (Crohn Colitis
  Diletants)
Jirovcova 24
37004 Ceske Budejovice
Budweis
Tel: +420 (0)3 83 83 89
Fax: +420 (0)3 83 84 47
ccd@volny.cz
www.volny.cz/ccd/

Denmark
Colitis–Crohn Foreningen (CCF)
Birkegrade 11
2200 København N
Tel: +45 (0)35 35 4882/4782
ccf@ccf.dk
www.ccf.dk

Europe

European Federation of Crohn's
and Ulcerative Colitis
Associations (EFCCA)
c/o Tor Erik Jorgensen
Parallellen 13A
N-1430 As
Norway
Tel: +47 (0)64 94 16 71
Fax: +47 (0)22 93 72 13
efcca@hotmail.com
www.efcca.org

Finland

Crohn Ja Colitis Ry (CCAFIN)
Kuninkaankatu 24 A, 2 krs
33210 Tampere
Tel: +358 (0)3 266 1489
Fax: +358 (0)20 482 2290
ccafin@sci.fi
www.sci.fi/~ccafin

France

Association François Aupetit
(AFA)
Hôpital Saint-Antoine
184 rue du Faubourg Saint-
Antoine
75012 Paris
Tel: +33 (0)1 43 07 00 49
www.afa.asso.fr
info@afa.asso.fr

Germany

Deutsche Morbus Crohn/Colitis
Ulcerosa-Vereinigung eV
Paracelsusstraße 15
51375 Leverkusen
Tel: +49 (0)214 87608 0
Fax: +49 (0)214 87608 88
info@dccv.de
www.dccv.de

Hungary

Magyarországi Crohn-Coliteses
Betegek Egyesülete (MCCBE)
Igmándi utca 22. Fzst. 1.
1112 Budapest
Tel: +36 (0)1 322 80 98
Fax: +36 (0)1 322 92 87
Tel (secretariat):
+36 (0)1 270 06 38
www.extra.hu/mccbe/
sternp@mav.hu

Ireland

Irish Society For Colitis and
Crohn's Disease (ISCC)
Carmichael Centre
North Brunswick Street
Dublin 7
Tel: +353 (0)1 872 1416
Fax: +353 (0)1 873 5737
info@iscc.ie
www.iscc.ie

Italy

Federazione Nazionale delle
 Associazione per la Malattie
 Infiammatorie Croniche dell'
 Intestino (AMICI)
Via A Wildt 19/4
20131 Milano
Tel: +39 02 28 93 673
Fax: +39 02 268 22 670
info@amiciitalia.org
www.amiciitalia.org

Luxembourg

Association Luxembourgeoise de
 la Maladie de Crohn (ALMC)
PO Box 648
2016 Luxembourg
Tel: +352 (0)50 98 28
Fax: +352 (0)47 98 20 20
rene.manderscheid@airport.
 etat.lu
www.afa.asso.fr/luxembourg/

Netherlands

Crohn En Colitis Ulcerosa
 Vereniging Nederland
Wilhelminastraat 45
3621 VG Breukelen
Tel: +31 (0)346 26 10 01
Fax: +31 (0)346 26 49 74
info@crohn-colitis.nl
www.crohn-colitis.nl

Norway

Landsforeningen MOT
 Fordøyelsessykdommer (LMF)
c/o FFO, Smågruppesekretariatet
Postboks 4568 Torshov
0404 Oslo
Tel: +47 (0)88 00 50 21
Fax: +47 (0)88 00 50 31
imfnorge@online.no
www.lmfnorge.no

Portugal

Associaçao Portuguesa da
 Doença Inflamatória do
 Intestino (APDI)
Rua Santa Catarina, n° 922 - 4°
 Esq.
4000-446 Porto
Tel: +351 22 208 6350
apdi@net.sapo.pt
www.apdi.org.pt

Slovakia

Slovak Crohn Club (SCC)
Malé námestie 28
901 01 Malacky
www.crohnclub.sk
crohnclub@crohnclub.sk/

South Africa

South African Crohn's & Colitis
  Association
PO Box 798
Fourways, 2055
Tel: +27 (0)11 465 7449
mossy@cybertrade.co.za
www.ccsg.org.za/ccsg.htm

Spain

Asociación de Enfermos de
  Crohn y Colitis Ulcerosa de
  España (ACCU)
C/ Hileras 4 - 4ª planta
Despachos 6 y 7
28013 Madrid
Tel: +34 (0)91 542 63 26 /
+34 (0)91 547 55 05
Fax: +34 (0)91 542 63 26
accuesp@accuesp.com
www.accuesp.com

Sweden

Riksförbundet för Mag- och
  Tarmsjuka (RMT)
Box 20054
104 60 Stockholm
Tel: +46 (0)8 642 42 00
Fax: +46 (0)8 642 11 00
rmt@magotarm.se
www.magotarm.se

Switzerland

Schweizerische Morbus
  Crohn/Colitis Ulcerosa-
  Vereinigung
Association Suisse de la Maladie
  de Crohn et Colite ulcéreuse
Associazione Svizzera Morbo di
  Crohn/Colite ulcerosa
Postfach
5001 Aarau
Tel/fax: +41 (0)62 824 87 07
(Tues 8–11 AM)
welcome@smccv.ch
www.smccv.ch / www.asmcc.ch

UK

National Association for Colitis
  and Crohn's disease (NACC)
4 Beaumont House
Sutton Road
St Albans
Hertfordshire AL1 5HH
Tel (administration): +44 (0)1727
  830038
Tel (information): +44 (0)1727
  844296 / 0845 130 2233
Fax: +44 (0)1727 862550
nacc@nacc.org.uk
www.nacc.org.uk

Ileostomy and Internal Pouch
  Support Group
Peverill House
1–5 Mill Road
Ballyclare, Co. Antrim
BT39 9DR
Tel: +44 (0)28 9334 4043 /
  0800 0184 724
Fax: +44 (0)28 9332 4606
info@the-ia.org.uk
www.the-ia.org.uk

USA

Crohn's and Colitis Foundation
  of America
386 Park Avenue South
17th Floor
New York NY 10016-8804
Tel: +1 212 685 3440 /
  1 800 932 2423
Fax: +1 212 779 4098
info@ccfa.org
www.ccfa.org

Further websites
www.ibdforum.com
ibd.patientcommunity.com
www.ibdclub.org.uk
www.gastrohep.com

Books
Allan RN, Rhodes JM,
Hanauer SB et al., eds.
Inflammatory Bowel Diseases,
3rd edn. New York: Churchill
Livingstone, 1997.

Greig ER, Rampton DS.
Management of Crohn's Disease.
London: Martin Dunitz, 2003.

Kirsner JB, Shorter RG, eds.
Inflammatory Bowel Disease, 4th
edn. Philadelphia: Lea & Febiger,
1995.

Stein SH, Hanauer SB, Rood RP,
Crohn's and Colitis Foundation
of America. *Inflammatory Bowel
Disease: A Guide for Patients
and Their Families*, 2nd edn.
Philadelphia: Lippincott Williams
and Wilkins, 1998.

Targan SR, Shanahan F,
Karp LC, eds. *Inflammatory
Bowel Disease. From Bench to
Bedside*, 2nd edn. Dordrecht:
Kluwer Academic Publishers,
2003.

Index

CD, Crohn's disease; UC, ulcerative colitis. Only information specific to CD or UC is indexed under those entry terms.

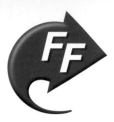

Imagine if every time you wanted to know something you knew where to look...

Over one million copies sold

- Written by world experts
- Concise and practical
- Up to date
- Designed for ease of reading and reference
- Copiously illustrated with useful photographs, diagrams and charts.

Our aim is to make *Fast Facts* **the world's most respected medical handbook series**. Feedback on how to make titles even more useful is always welcome (feedback@fastfacts.com).

Over 70 *Fast Facts* titles, including:

Asthma
Benign Gynecological Disease (second edition)
Benign Prostatic Hyperplasia (fifth edition)
Bipolar Disorder
Bladder Cancer
Bleeding Disorders
Brain Tumors
Breast Cancer (third edition)
Celiac Disease
Chronic Obstructive Pulmonary Disease
Colorectal Cancer (second edition)
Contraception (second edition)
Dementia
Depression (second edition)
Dyspepsia (second edition)
Eczema and Contact Dermatitis
Endometriosis (second edition)
Epilepsy (third edition)
Erectile Dysfunction (third edition)
Gynecological Oncology
Headaches (second edition)

Hyperlipidemia (third edition)
Hypertension (second edition)
Irritable Bowel Syndrome (second edition)
Menopause (second edition)
Minor Surgery
Multiple Sclerosis (second edition)
Ophthalmology
Osteoporosis (fourth edition)
Parkinson's Disease
Prostate Cancer (fourth edition)
Psoriasis (second edition)
Respiratory Tract Infection (second edition)
Rheumatoid Arthritis
Schizophrenia (second edition)
Sexual Dysfunction
Sexually Transmitted Infections
Skin Cancer
Smoking Cessation
Soft Tissue Rheumatology
Thyroid Disorders
Urinary Stones

Orders

To order via the website, or to find regional distributors, please go to www.fastfacts.com

For telephone orders, please call +44 (0)1752 202301 (Europe), 1 800 247 6553 (USA, toll free) or +1 419 281 1802 (Americas)